Praise for *Solving the Weight Loss Puzzle*

"How do you spell healthy, sane, and safe weight loss? P-L-O-U-R-D-E! I love Dr. Plourdé, and his book will transform your body, your thinking and your life!"
—*New York Times* bestselling author Michael Levin

"In this book, Dr. Plourdé offers us a multi-parametric approach to a puzzle and indeed dilemma affecting many of us—and that is the problem of obesity and the weight loss struggle. His approach which encompasses human biochemistry, physiology, exercise science, and faith provides a solution which not only WILL work, but also results in a transformation of health and well being for those who adhere to the METHOD. His conversational style and clarity makes the information in this work both approachable and useful on a practical basis. Begin!!"
—Allan M. Haggar, M.D.

"This book is a wonderful compilation of Dr. Plourdé's years of laboratory research. He has worked tirelessly to pursue the most up to date science. *Solving The Weight Loss Puzzle* details not only his compassion, but also his intensely focused professional goals to perfect "The Plourdé Method". I want to congratulate Dr. Plourdé on another major accomplishment in his work to support individuals wishing to be successful with their weight loss efforts."
— Kathleen Rourke, B.S., B.S.N., M.S., Ph.D., M.S.N., R.N., RD

Solving the Weight Loss Puzzle

The Plourdé Method℠

Solving the Weight Loss Puzzle

DAVID B. PLOURDÉ, Ph.D.

Copyright © 2024

All rights reserved. This book or any portion thereof may not be reproduced or used in any manner whatsoever without the express written permission of the author except for the use of brief quotations in a book review.

ISBN (paperback): 979-8-218-49939-6
ISBN (ebook): 979-8-218-53136-2

Book design and production by www.AuthorSuccess.com
Cover art by iStock

Printed in the United States of America

Disclaimer

Dr. Plourdé is a Ph.D. level scientist in the fields of human nutrition and exercise physiology. He is not a medical doctor. Significant body fat weight loss may have physiological implications on your need for medications. This must be taken seriously. Always consult your personal medical doctor in these matters.

Book Dedication

I dedicate this book to my late brother, Bill Plourdé. Bill was my best friend. He was my mentor. He was my goal: I wanted to be just like him. He was not only one of the strongest people I've ever known, but more importantly, he was one of the most kind, generous, and unselfish human beings that I have ever encountered. He inspired my faith in the Savior, Jesus Christ. He inspired me to become an elite athlete—which later translated into a passion for physical sciences. I owe so much to my brother for all of his Christ-like qualities that helped me to become the man that I am today. In fact, I wouldn't be writing this to you right now if it were not for him.

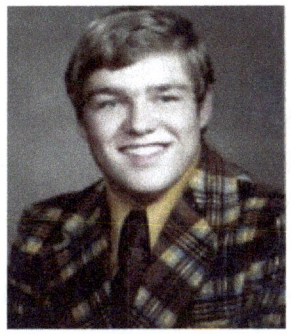

Bill's high school senior photo
Source: Plourdé family photo

This is where it gets personal: my brother struggled with being overweight and was challenged with many of the associated diseases that go along with it.

A secret that I am now willing to share with my readers is that among the thousands of people who I've worked with in my professional career, my brother was, perhaps, the one person I wanted to help the most, but he waited too long. He became a type II diabetic and had developed a non-alcoholic fatty liver. The cumulative years of insulin injection, hyperinsulinemia, and inflammation lead to severe heart disease, and he sadly passed away on my birthday in 2013, at the early age of fifty-five, from a sudden massive heart attack. This is a very sad truth for me. There isn't a day that goes by that I don't think about my brother. I love him, miss him, and seek to honor him in writing this book. The silver lining is that although I was not able to help my brother the way that I had hoped, perhaps I may be able to help you.

In 2019, God blessed my wife Tiffany and I with a son in my later life. As you might have anticipated, he is named after both my brother and my father—both were named William and both have since passed away. On a side note, the name William means "the protector;" very fitting for two of the most important men in my life.

Our son William is truly a blessing from God. I'm also so incredibly blessed to also have four amazing daughters: Briana is a neuroscientist, Sophia is an exercise scientist (and helps me run The Plourdé Institute), Venessa is pursuing psychology and is considering becoming a Doctor of Psychology, and my fourth daughter Alana is the artist among us and will be entering film school in the fall of this year.

My ultimate hope is that the ideas in this book will liberate you from the struggle of food addiction, obesity, and disease and help to bring you into a new life of freedom, better health, joy, and self-respect.

Here's to your success!

Contents

Intended Audience		xi
Why Should You Read This Book?		xiii
A Word to the Reader		xv
Chapter 1	How Did I Get Here?	1
Chapter 2	A Scientific Breakthrough	5
Chapter 3	A Strange Observation: Jennifer's Unexplained Weight Loss Plateau	9
Chapter 4	The Day Everything Changed	18
Chapter 5	The Research Continues! A Scientific Explanation for Your Weight Loss Plateau	24
Chapter 6	If Your Fat Cells Could Talk, They'd Say: "ABSOLUTELY NOT!"	35
Chapter 7	The Most Crucial Puzzle Piece: Your Meal Plan	49
	Subsection: Seven Factors to Prevent Constipation in Your Weight Loss Journey	68
	Subsection: Avoid the Pitfall of Salt Spikes and Water Retention	76
Chapter 8	I Hate to Break the Bad News . . .	85
Chapter 9	Everything You Think You Know About Exercise Is Wrong!	101
Chapter 10	The Dark Side of Semaglutide Medications	126
	Subsection: The Plourde Method^{SM}— A Healthy Alternative to Semaglutide Medications	136

Chapter 11	Are You Ready to Be Accountable?	139
Chapter 12	Your Body Fat, Your Health, and Disease	150
	Subsection: Understanding Inflammation	165
Chapter 13	When Food is Your Drug	176
Chapter 14	Confessions of a Weight Loss Counselor	203
Chapter 15	The Power of Faith	213
Chapter 16	The Keys to Long Term Weight Loss Success	219
Chapter 17	A Personal Invitation from Dr. Plourdé	228
Acknowledgments		231
Bibliography		234

Intended Audience

This book is written for untrained to moderately trained overweight adult men and women. This is not a vegetarian or vegan diet. This book is *not intended for nutritional or exercise guidance for elite athletes or people who are in excellent physical condition.*

Why Should You Read This Book?

For thirty-three years, David Plourdé, Ph.D., has observed and guided thousands of overweight individuals in a human performance laboratory. He developed a scientific weight loss method based on these studies, and dedicated his life to refining it. Dr. Plourdé realized very early on that successful weight loss must involve *the unique integration of advanced physical sciences, the psychology of eating behavior, and faith.*

When you think about it, weight loss has probably been a complex and frustrating puzzle for you. The goal of this book is to provide you with all of the puzzle pieces and put them in their proper place, thus finally putting an end to your painful frustration and confusion. Some of the puzzle pieces this book will help you to identify are:

1. Fat Cells: How do they work and what are some of the *unseen* roadblocks that prevent you from successful weight loss (which really means fat loss)?
2. What dietary regimen is the most effective for weight loss?
3. What type of exercise is the most effective for weight loss?
4. How does understanding your psychology and emotional intelligence factor into successful weight loss?

5. Why is personal accountability so necessary for successful weight loss?
6. What if I have a food addiction? Can I still be successful in my weight loss journey?
7. What is faith and why could it be a missing piece in your weight loss puzzle?

There has never been a book written like this before. There has never been a weight loss program like this before. If you apply the principles outlined here, you can expect to replace the psychological, emotional, and physical pain of obesity—and its associated diseases—with a new life marked by freedom, better health, joy, and self-respect.

A Word to the Reader

Throughout my career, I've served highly successful CEOs, board chairmen and women, business owners, and leaders in every field to help them accomplish the one thing that they couldn't do on their own: successful weight loss. Up until now, the information contained in this book has only been available to the affluent; those who could afford to invest in this important, but resource-intensive, act of self-care. For a time, I have felt a moral obligation to write this book and make the principles of THE PLOURDE METHOD℠ available to everyone, including you, personally.

Having said that, the road map I have laid out in this book *is not the full breadth of intellectual property and trade secrets* that I've accumulated over the past decades, but it does include the heart of the METHOD. People who embrace and carefully follow these principles may experience a 50 percent reduction from their peak body fat weight. For many of you, your peak body fat weight is now; for others, it may have occurred during pregnancy; for some, your highest body fat occurred at some other point in the past. Regardless, this version of THE PLOURDE METHOD℠ will allow the body to tolerate a 50 percent reduction from peak body fatness, without any threat to metabolic homeostasis (the brain's perception of metabolic stability).

The full extent of intellectual property and trade secrets of THE

PLOURDE METHOD℠ are made available to only the private clients of The Plourdé Institute. If, after reading this book, you desire exposure to the entire methodology, you will learn how to reach out to us in the Personal Invitation chapter. Let me assure you that if you are unable to engage with me personally, I wrote this book for you. In fact, I had you in mind every moment of this arduous journey. Trust me, writing is *not* my wheelhouse. This was truly a labor of love. I've got you.

Best Wishes, D.P.

CHAPTER 1

How Did I Get Here?

▶▶▶ As a teenager, I was a three-time state champion competitive powerlifter and set numerous state records. I was coached by Bill Seno, a world champion, author, and dear friend. All my peers that I trained with were world champions. It was truly an honor and privilege for me to even be in their presence. I was expected to be a world champion eventually, and I fully accepted that as my path.

Succeeding in sports was fun and exhilarating. I had tremendous confidence in myself, but I also had a major problem that no one really even knew about: I suffered from exercise-induced hypoglycemia, which is low blood sugar caused by excessive exercise. It was so severe that it affected my vision. I could barely read. I couldn't stay awake. My reading comprehension was terrible and my grades in school testified to that fact. I survived school by charming my teachers. My teachers liked me, and they graciously helped me along my academic journey (although I'm not so sure I deserved it). I graduated from high school with a GPA of 1.9 and I got into college on academic probation because I could play football. As a freshman in college, I was the strongest athlete on the football team.

As I progressed through college, my training became more and more extreme, resulting in greater instability with my blood sugar. At that time, I had a girlfriend who was a gymnast at the

University of Michigan. I would drive to see her from time to time and it was a miracle for me to get back alive. I literally could *not* stay awake. It was chronic and I didn't understand why I was suffering this way.

That all changed my junior year in college when my sister Loree gave me my first book on nutrition science. My sister was the chief information officer (CIO) of one of the largest insurance companies in the world and was always a straight-A student. She knew I was struggling, and her loving act of sharing that book was a game changer. The essence of the book proposed a low to moderate protein, moderate fat, high fiber diet (consisting of mostly vegetables) absent of obvious sugars. This was coupled with gentle aerobic exercise, and this combination proved to be beneficial on so many levels! Of course, reading the book was very difficult. I had to force myself to stay awake as I read and reread every chapter, feverishly applying every syllable of the book.

What happened next changed my life forever. My vision and reading comprehension improved almost immediately. My mental acuity was sharp as a tack. I was no longer constantly drowsy and had no problem staying focused while I drove my vehicle or studied. In a matter of months, my grades went from very poor to a 4.0. My professors started to say things to me like, "When you get into your career, you need to remember the poor."

I would look both ways and wonder who the heck they were talking to! Certainly, people would always affirm me for my athletic prowess, but for a professor to tell me that I was incredibly smart and had a bright future professionally was completely foreign to me. The truth is that it was shocking, but I actually believed it, which, unbeknownst to me, was a principle of faith (which we will talk about in a later chapter)! This was a defining moment for me. I made an immediate about face: I abruptly quit competitive powerlifting *and* playing college football. My sole focus became my academics and I've never looked back since that day.

As I was wrapping up my undergraduate degree at the University of Wisconsin-Whitewater, I was required to design an internship. I proposed to the college that I run a weight loss program for overweight college students. Since I was an athlete with a background in exercise physiology and human performance, and now was headlong pursuing nutrition science and chemistry, they said, "Why not?" The university was kind enough to advertise my program in the university newspaper. Before I knew it, I had a full caseload of clients.

On the first day, I walked into the university health center and then into my private office that overlooked the campus. I sat down behind the desk, looked up, and said a prayer, "Thank you, God!," because I knew this wasn't going to be just an internship, it was a spiritual awakening about the new calling and direction for my life in science. My internship gave me the opportunity to personally teach overweight college students sound principles of nutrition and eating behavior, as well as exercise physiology. Their outcomes were profound: significant body fat weight loss occurred across the board, along with greater energy, mental acuity, and improved self-esteem. I realized the impact I was having was meaningful to them, but also very gratifying to me professionally.

Throughout my college experience, I also led two campus ministries: InterVarsity Christian Fellowship and Fellowship of Christian Athletes. I had chosen social work as a major because I knew I would learn therapeutic counseling skills that would come in handy later in what I believed at that time was my calling: to go into Christian ministry full-time. However, my life was so profoundly improved by the principles I had learned in nutrition science and exercise physiology, coupled with feelings of such professional gratification, that I knew seminary was not the answer for me.

I completed my undergraduate degree in 1989, and founded my business, The Plourdé Institute, formally in 1991. Not long after this, I matriculated into a Ph.D. program where I could receive doctoral credentials in more than one field at the same time: a feat that literally almost killed me (only half joking). ▶▶▶

As I conclude this first segment, I cannot overstate the significance of the pain that I endured and perhaps the greater purpose the pain served me in shaping my life. I truly believe that without it, I would never have gotten here. The remainder of these chapters will outline the arduous path that I undertook to learn the principles that I am about to teach you.

As you journey with me, I want you to be particularly mindful of the pain that you are feeling right now: perhaps your pain is insecurity, shame, embarrassment, self-loathing, fear, frustration, or even confusion. Is it possible that channeling your pain towards a sound, interdisciplinary, and scientific solution may be *the necessary ingredient that you've overlooked*?

The strange truth that I have observed over my entire career is that every successful weight loss experience has *always begun with a high level of pain*. When people reach out to me and ask for help, the first thing I do in the intake process is assess their clinical need for weight loss and also determine the level of pain they're experiencing. If a person's pain does not rise to a high enough threshold, my experience shows that they often don't have the psychological or emotional urgency for change needed for the journey. So, as you contemplate your own circumstances, realize this: if you are in a high level of pain, you're actually in good company and will likely have the psychological and emotional gas to climb this challenging terrain with me. Do you believe me? If so, take my hand and let's walk together . . .

CHAPTER 2

A Scientific Breakthrough

▶▶▶ In early September 1994, I was the first person in the world to purchase an instrument called the BOD POD. It was an incredible breakthrough in the field of weight loss because prior to 1994, the only accurate way to measure fat and lean tissue in the human body was to dunk people underwater: it's called hydrostatic weighing, and it was an arduous, stressful, and often inaccurate way to measure human body composition.

I would take my clients to the Wheaton College (IL) human performance laboratory, where clients would undergo the testing. With the help of scientist Glenn Town, Ph.D., Chair of the Department of Exercise Physiology, we would assess body composition accurately. However, the process was not only stressful and potentially dangerous, but it was also embarrassing for my clients.

It required them to wear a skimpy bathing suit, to climb up a ladder, then to be fully submerged in a large tank of water without any air in their lungs while we measured how much they weighed underwater. My clients hated the process, and it was almost impossible to get them to come back for repeat testing. This would definitely be a problem for a weight loss business, wouldn't it? LOL.

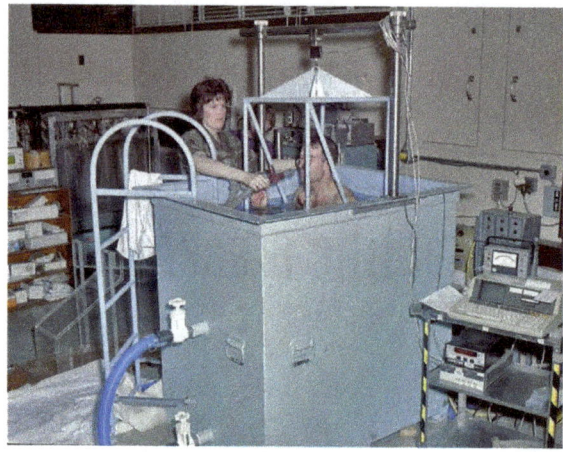

Hydrostatic Weighing Lab
Photo Source: Public Domain

When the BOD POD came to market in 1994, it was a complete departure from traditional body composition testing, because rather than using water to measure the volume of the body, the BOD POD used air displacement. Not a single person, institution, or sports team was willing to take the risk on such a novel approach to measuring body fat.

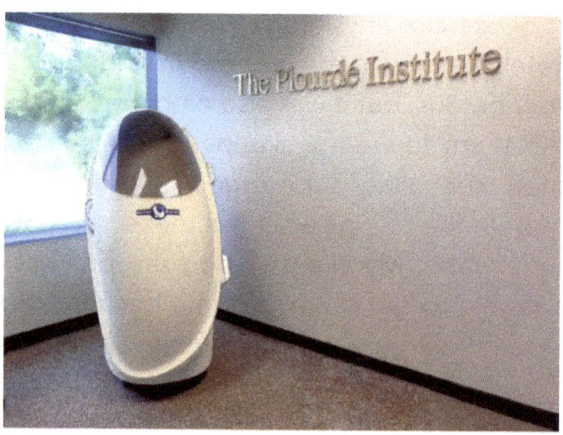

Credit: The Plourdé Institute

That's when I met with one of the co-inventors, Susan Aitkens, M.S., at the American College of Sports Medicine convention in Indianapolis, Indiana. I drove five hours from where I lived in the western Chicago suburbs, and intended to be tested in the BOD POD. When I arrived, Susan told me that she was not testing anybody, but rather just showing people the device. I explained to her that I was dead set on getting tested and that there would be no consideration of a purchase if I didn't get measured. She agreed.

On that fateful day, she measured me in the BOD POD, and I realized that *this* was the breakthrough I was looking for: a method of measuring human body composition in a manner that was NOT stressful, completely safe, and *very accurate.* We quickly agreed on a purchase price, and the first BOD POD ever purchased was delivered to the Institute in Lisle, Illinois, in September 1994.

To promote the BOD POD, Life Measurement Instruments, the original creator of the BOD POD, organized a national media campaign, where journalists interviewed me and the segment aired on ABC, CBS, and NBC networks nationwide. That was a really cool moment! Shortly after that, in 1995, the strength coach of the Buffalo Bills, Rusty Jones, along with other team staff flew to Chicago for me to explain the physics of the BOD POD and how to use it. Needless to say, they were more than impressed and quickly purchased a BOD POD for their NFL team. Today, all college football players seeking to enter the NFL at the NFL Combine undergo body composition testing with the BOD POD as a prerequisite in their assessments of athletes. I feel truly humbled to be part of that story. ▶▶▶

You might ask why I have spent so much time discussing the BOD POD. It's because for the first time in my career, I could measure very precise changes in body fat and lean tissue in overweight human subjects as they were going through their weight loss journey. Accumulating accurate body composition data was much easier because the test subjects were no longer stressed out by the experience. We NEVER looked back! I have personally conducted more measurements with the BOD POD than any other institution in the world.

CHAPTER 3

A Strange Observation: Jennifer's Unexplained Weight Loss Plateau

Everything changed when my client, Jennifer from Batavia, Illinois, entered the program. She was the first person I very carefully monitored in our science-based weight loss program using the BOD POD. Her weight loss outcome was eye-opening.

Let's dive into Jennifer's story.

▶▶▶ First, let me explain some of her backstory: she was succeeding in every area of her life except for one . . . she was overweight. She was well educated and held a master's degree in physical therapy. She was happily married and the mother of two beautiful kids. Jennifer should have been living her best life—but she was miserable in her skin. She was more than ready to learn and eager to cooperate. From the very beginning, we had great rapport. She thoroughly enjoyed the program and followed it to a T. At that time, THE PLOURDE METHOD® was a low to moderate protein, moderate fat, high fiber diet with the removal of all obvious sugars and starches. I coupled the diet with gentle aerobic exercise. It worked beautifully.

She arrived at the Institute on Monday, September 12, 1994. I conducted a half-day science-based weight loss assessment. She was thirty-six years old, 5 feet 2 ¼ inches tall, and weighed 220 pounds. She underwent body composition testing in the BOD POD. The test results revealed that she had 101 pounds of lean tissue while maintaining 119 pounds of body fat.

Through a very thorough health history interview process, we ascertained that at the age of sixteen, Jennifer had weighed approximately 120 pounds and maintained slightly low body fat at 18 percent of her total weight. This translated to 21.6 pounds of body fat and 98.4 pounds of lean tissue.

Her all-time highest body weight occurred at the age of thirty-one years old (after the birth of her second child) when she weighed 240 pounds. If we make the assumption that her lean tissue was approximately the same at the age of thirty-one years as it was when she was thirty-six years old—at 101 pounds, she would've maintained 139 pounds of body fat at her peak body fatness. This is an extrapolated data point, but it is significant.

If the assumption is accurate, she gained 117.4 pounds of body fat between the ages of sixteen and thirty-one years old. This would represent an approximately **543.5 percent increase in body fat since the age of sixteen**.

See the chart depicting the changes in Jennifer's body fat from the baseline of physical maturity:

The Plourdé Institute
An Interdisciplinary Science-Based Approach to Weight Loss

Historical Evaluation of Adiposity

Name _____Jennifer_____   Date _____9/12/1994_____

Condition of Adiposity	Baseline	Peak	Current	Goal - 50%
Body Fat %	18.0	57.9	54.1	40.3
Fat Weight	21.6	139.0	119.0	69.5
Lean Weight	98.4	101.0	101.0	103.0
Total Weight	120.0	240.0	220	172.5
Age	16	31	36	36
# of Adipocytes	16.3	52.5	52.5	52.5

Fat Weight Increase of ____117.4____ lbs. = ____543.5____ %

Type of Lipogenesis =

(Type 1) Adipocyte Hypertrophy ☐

(Type 2) Adipocyte Hyperplastic Hypertrophy (Both Types) ☐

Copyright © 2023 David Plourdé, Ph.D.

www.theplourdeinstitute.com
901 Warrenville Road, Suite 110, Lisle, Illinois, 60532   630.769.0776

Credit: The Plourdé Institute

12   Solving the Weight Loss Puzzle

Jennifer was measured approximately once every four weeks for twelve months beginning September 12 of 1994 through August of 1995. See the spreadsheet below for all of her body composition data, including the extrapolated data point dating back to 1989:

The Plourdé Institute
An Interdisciplinary Science-Based Approach to Weight Loss

| BODY COMPOSITION PROGRESS CHART ||||||||
| CLIENT NAME: JENNIFER ||| | GOAL FAT WEIGHT: 69.5 |||
DATE	TOTAL WEIGHT	FAT WEIGHT	LEAN WEIGHT	FAT LOSS	% FAT LOSS	TOTAL FAT LOSS
9/12/1989	240.0	139.0	101.0			
9/12/1994	220.0	119.0	101.0	20.00	-14.4%	20.00
10/7/1994	210.8	108.6	102.2	10.36	-8.7%	30.36
11/4/1994	197.6	94.7	102.9	13.88	-12.8%	44.24
12/30/1994	191.8	88.2	103.6	6.51	-6.9%	50.75
1/27/1995	180.6	76.4	104.2	11.83	-13.4%	62.58
3/17/1995	177.2	72.7	104.5	3.69	-4.8%	66.27
4/7/1995	173.9	68.8	105.1	3.89	-5.3%	70.16
6/9/1995	174.5	70.7	103.8	-1.93	+2.8%	68.23
7/7/1995	171.7	66.3	105.4	4.46	-6.3%	72.69
8/31/1995	168.0	64.2	103.8	2.08	-3.1%	74.76

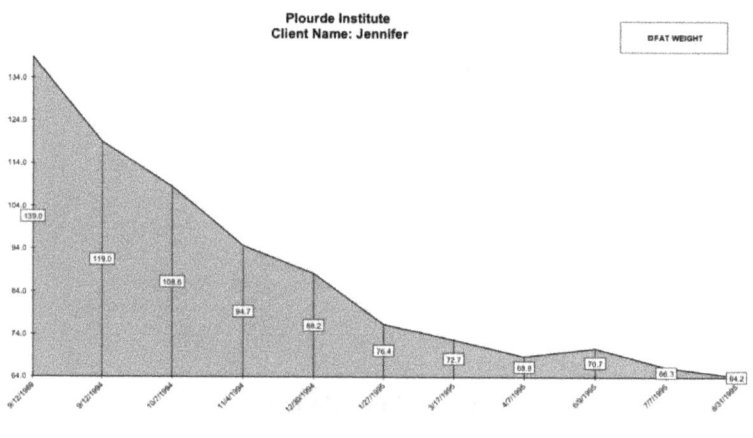

Credit: The Plourdé Institute

A Strange Observation: Jennifer's Unexplained Weight Loss Plateau

The *strange observation* that I made while tracking Jennifer occurred six months into her weight loss experience. Her body fat at the peak was 139 pounds, with a total weight of 240 pounds. At six months, her total weight had come down to 177.2 pounds and her body fat had reduced to 72.7 pounds. This was just shy of a 50 percent body fat weight loss. Strangely, no matter how regimented her diet and no matter how rigorous the exercise, there was no further substantial body fat weight loss at this point. After five months of stagnation, frustrated by the lack of progress, she quit the program. Let me mention that I was also very frustrated by this outcome. It was baffling to me that her body would not allow further fat loss. ▶▶▶

When you make an eye-opening observation *once*, it's interesting, but after making an observation hundreds of times, you are witnessing a phenomenon. As more people continued to come to the Institute, I kept seeing a very fascinating and frustrating pattern emerge: if a man had a peak body fat weight of one hundred pounds, once he hit approximately fifty pounds of fat, he would strangely stop losing. If a woman had eighty pounds of fat at her peak, she would stop losing at approximately forty pounds. There seemed to be a relatively hard stop at 50 percent body fat weight loss from the peak, regardless of gender. You get the picture. I thought to myself, "People should be able to lose more than 50 percent of their total body fat, shouldn't they?"

Well, frustrated, but equally fascinated by this strange pattern and also intrigued, I started to do literature searches. I came across a very obscure scientific paper published in 1971 entitled "Adipose Cellularity in Relation to Human Obesity" by Dr. Jules Hirsch (Hirsch, 1971). His research was groundbreaking. In the 1960s, he extracted fat cells from adults who had never been overweight and who had completely normal body fat levels. **He learned that normal fat cells weighed approximately .7 of a microgram.**

Adipocyte (Fat Cell)

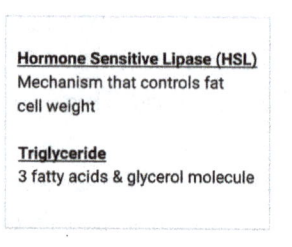
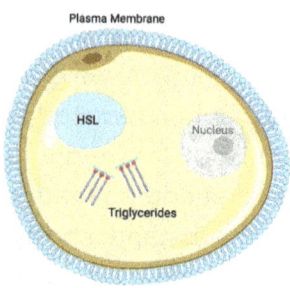

Hormone Sensitive Lipase (HSL)
Mechanism that controls fat cell weight

Triglyceride
3 fatty acids & glycerol molecule

Normal Fat Cell Weight:
0.7 micrograms

Credit: Created in BioRender. Plourde, D., Plourde, B. (2024) BioRender.com/m65f625

If you're not a science person, you probably don't have a frame of reference for what one microgram is. So let me give you one: a one-liter bottle of water weighs exactly 2.205 pounds or one kilogram (a metric unit for weight). One microgram is a billionth of a kilogram. Fat cells are very small!

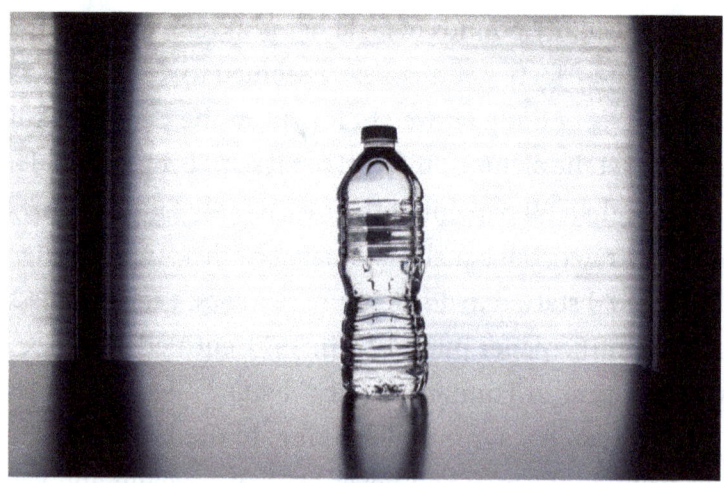

1 Liter Bottle of Water weighs 1 Kilogram or 2.205 pounds.
Credit: Steve Johnson on Unsplash

Dr. Hirsch went on to extract fat cells from people who were clinically obese at their highest body fat levels. What he learned was absolutely remarkable: the heaviest fat cells ever measured in overweight human subjects was approximately 1.4 micrograms. In other words, **the heaviest fat cells were double the weight of a normal weight fat cell. Conversely, normal fat cells were half the weight of the very largest fat cells.**

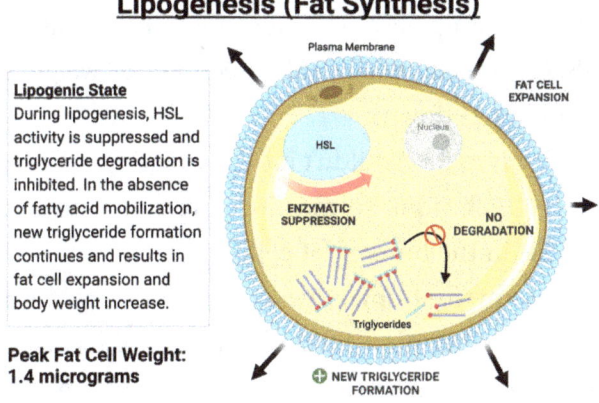

Credit: Created in BioRender. Plourde, D., Plourde, B. (2024) BioRender.com/b68u802

*At that moment, the lights went on for me. What I theorized regarding Jennifer's experience in 1994 was simply this: her fat cells went from 1.4 micrograms while at 139 pounds of fat and reduced to .7 of a microgram at what seemed to be a natural biological plateau at nearly 70 pounds of fat—**approximately 50 percent less body fat.***

I asked myself, "Could it be that her body resisted further fat loss when her fat cells resumed to a normal weight? Is it possible that the body was preventing additional fat loss because the body perceived a threat to her metabolic homeostasis (metabolic stability) if fat loss continued?" I would have to research this formally to find out.

> **FACT: The enzyme Hormone-Sensitive Lipase (later abbreviated throughout the book as HSL) regulates fat cell weight: it determines whether fat cells get bigger or smaller.**

When fat cells get bigger, it's because new storage fat is being created in the cell (it's called triglyceride). When fat cells get heavier, body fat weight goes up because body fat weight is simply the weight of all fat cells. Conversely, when HSL directs fat cell weight to decrease, body fat weight goes down.

I thought to myself, "Wouldn't it be interesting if I could develop a non-invasive technique to monitor the function of Hormone-Sensitive Lipase in the human fat cell?"

This became my first objective as a scientist, and I achieved it in August of 2000 after monitoring hundreds of human subjects at the Institute. I examined closely the underlying chemical quality of foods, fluids, and products and correlated them to precise changes in fuel utilization in cellular work (whether the body used fat, sugar, or protein to drive cellular metabolism).

Highly motivated by these findings, I matriculated into the Ph.D. program at Union Institute and University in Cincinnati, Ohio. After entering my doctoral research program, my next question was, "Wouldn't it be interesting if I could develop a full scientific methodology to control the enzyme HSL?"

I was able to accomplish my second objective, but only after I tracked 308 adult obese human subjects divided among three trials while answering to the Institutional Review Board. This requirement is a safeguard for the safe and ethical treatment of human subjects in research.

My third and final objective was to select and establish a statistical tool that would predict when the human body would resist fat loss biologically and naturally plateau. After the three trials were completed and a thorough statistical analysis was conducted, my final objective was complete. It was at this point that, with the help of Dr. Brad Lindell, we chose the **95 percent confidence interval** to become the tool to predict such an outcome.

My ultimate goal was to provide an interdisciplinary science-based weight loss solution founded on the most advanced methods in nutrition science, exercise physiology, human body composition science, and the psychology of eating behavior, as well as food addiction recovery.

What I learned from my research was absolutely mind blowing. I know that as a scientist, I'm supposed to be more stoic, but I know what's up ahead for you if you apply these principles, and I am so excited for you! This information will help you put all of the pieces of the proverbial weight loss puzzle in place and help replace your frustration and confusion with clarity, hope, and motivation.

Are you with me? Let's keep this rolling!

CHAPTER 4

The Day Everything Changed

▶▶▶ This story begins on June 1, 2000, when Vince from Naperville, Illinois, came in for a half-day science-based weight loss assessment. He was a sixty-six-year-old CEO of a large homebuilding company with expertise in sales and marketing. We placed Vince in the BOD POD and learned that his total weight was 259.3 pounds, his body fat weight was 124 pounds, and his lean weight was 135.3 pounds. This was the most Vince had ever weighed in his life. In his intake process, we had pre-determined that he had a high clinical need for weight loss and was psychologically and emotionally ready for change. Vince and I had a great rapport, and I found him to be very receptive and enthusiastic. He decisively moved forward with the program.

At his onboarding, I gave him a full explanation of the METHOD (what it was at that time). This entailed a low-to-moderate protein, moderate fat, high-fiber diet. At least half of the meals were vegetables free of naturally occurring sugars and starches. Calorie targets, specific meal plan, exercise prescription, a daily logging system, and a structure of consistent accountability were provided. Vince came in for weekly visits where we measured his total body weight, conducted metabolic measurement testing, reviewed his overall program compliance, and concluded by setting specific behavioral goals. He was very excited about the progress he was seeing.

We measured him in the BOD POD every four weeks, and we observed continuous reduction in fat weight, which was very encouraging to him. It's a fact that over the course of my career I've served some highly educated and super successful individuals. I've had the benefit of learning from these people about things that they've uncovered in their chosen fields. My experience with Vince was no exception. He was an authority in sales and marketing and it was an honor to work with him.

I thought, wouldn't it be cool if I could take him out for lunch and pick his brain regarding pearls of wisdom about sales and marketing? So, on August 24 of the same year, at the close of one of our sessions, I asked him for a favor. I said, "Would you mind if I took you out for lunch and asked you some questions about what you've learned in sales and marketing? I'd love to pick your brain and grow in my own knowledge."

He happily agreed. So, on the following Thursday, I took Vince to a very high-end restaurant because of course he was Mr. VIP. Just kidding—I took him to a popular national sandwich chain restaurant.

As we were in line, he followed the teacher. I had a salad with lettuce, cucumbers, and chicken breast with some cheese sprinkled on top and oil and vinegar as my dressing. He did exactly as I did. We quickly sat down and ate our delicious salads and I began to pelt him with a series of questions about key lessons that he had learned in sales and marketing over his long career as a top executive. He was very generous, and if you don't know me, I'm a copious notetaker. I carefully wrote down every word Vince shared.

We concluded our lunch meeting and went straight to the Institute for his weekly session. I need you to understand something. Vince was recording every morsel of food and every ounce of fluid in a detailed nutrition and exercise log that I provided for him, so I had a full record of everything Vince had consumed that week. The only thing I didn't know for sure is what the heck we had just eaten at the sandwich shop.

We began his session with a weekly weight check and then proceeded to our human performance laboratory, where we conducted metabolic measurement testing. Given Vince's close adherence to the program, I would've expected for him to have a high rate of fat utilization. Much to my astonishment, I saw the exact opposite: very little fat was being utilized and the predominant source of fuel was glucose. I scratched my head, baffled by my observation. Everything that Vince had consumed for the week, as well as the nature of his eating and drinking behavior, was on target.

So, a lightbulb went on! I figured maybe there was something peculiar or different about what we ate at lunch. So, I picked up the phone and called the owner of that local franchise. She answered and I said, "Hi! My name is David and I was just at the restaurant and had a delicious fresh salad made up of lettuce, chicken, a sprinkle of cheese, some cucumber, and oil and vinegar." I proceeded to speak on Vince's behalf. I said, "I just left the restaurant and thank you so much for the great food and amazing experience today that my friend and I enjoyed. But I do have to tell you that I'm experiencing what I think is an adverse reaction to the meal."

I went on to say, "I think my blood sugar is elevated and I thought I would call you and ask you some questions about the details of the contents of my meal. Let me assure you, I'm not angry, I'm not in danger, and I have no ill motive. I just simply want to know some details about my meal."

I explained that my physician had pressed me to be more careful in managing my blood sugar. Once I learned the details of the meal, I would simply alter what I ordered so I could be more careful to comply with my physician's instructions the next time I visited.

She responded, "No problem."

I asked her, "Could you please tell me the ingredients of the chicken that I ate that was on my salad?"

She said, "I'd be happy to."

She put me on hold and went back to the kitchen, opened up the refrigerator, and found the cardboard box that contained the chicken and proceeded to tear off the portion with the ingredients. She brought it back to the telephone and kindly recited the list to me. I was expecting to hear: chicken breast, salt, spices. Nope. What came next turned the lights on.

She read: chicken meat, water, modified food starch, and a whole list of spices and preservatives. The ingredient that grabbed my attention was modified food starch. What I learned on that fateful day was that although the chicken we ate was quite tasty, it was technically not pure chicken, but rather a chicken product engineered to look like a chicken breast. The dirty little secret here is that the product was laced with modified food starch, which is a code phrase for corn flour.

In other words, that chicken was **not** chicken. It was a chicken product containing a filler that reduces the cost of protein by weight. The problem here is that it looked, smelled, and tasted like normal chicken. So, when a diabetic consumes that product, they would be unaware that their blood sugar is likely to go up with an impending secretion of insulin or a greater need for insulin.

My conversation with the restaurant owner continued. I said, "Thank you so much. Since I have you on the phone, can I trouble you to ask for the ingredients of the cheese that was sprinkled over my salad?"

She agreed and went back to the kitchen and retrieved the ingredients for the shredded cheddar cheese. Once back on the phone, she read the ingredients list.

What I was expecting was typical cheese ingredients: milk, salt, enzymes, and in some cases, color. When she began to recite the ingredients list, *again* the lights went on. The ingredients were: milk, salt, powdered cellulose, enzymes, and color. I said to myself, "Wait a minute? Powdered cellulose? What is powdered cellulose and why is it in the cheese?"

So, I quickly searched in one of my reference books and learned that powdered cellulose is a code phrase for potato flour. It can also be called potato starch, as well as microcrystalline cellulose. I realized that the cheese that was sprinkled on my salad was not normal cheese, but in fact, it was pre-shredded and the insidious potato flour was added as an anti-caking agent.

I later learned that if the manufacturing process involves the cheese being pre-shredded, cubed, or crumbled, it will contain this little-known ingredient. Apparently, cheese manufacturers have been including this ingredient for years to improve processing efficiency. Without it, cheese would get stuck in the slicing mechanisms and halt the manufacturing process.

Here again, the problem was that Vince and I sat down to eat a low to moderate protein, moderate fat, and high-fiber meal that we believed to be absent of sugar and starch. What I quickly realized was that there were insidious carbohydrates in the chicken as well as the cheese! I told the woman, "This information has been invaluable to me. Thank you so much! Can I trouble you for one more thing?"

Again, she agreed since it was late afternoon and the restaurant was slow. I asked her for the ingredients list of the oil and vinegar recipe. Once she got it, she came back to the phone to share it with me. By this point, I was suspicious, but I was still hoping for her to read the following: oil, vinegar, and spices. Well, I bet you guessed it—that's not what the ingredients list was. The ingredients list included the following: oil, vinegar, spices, and three forms of added sugar.

When I heard the ingredients list of the oil and vinegar recipe and had processed all of the information that she had just shared in a matter of minutes, it was a defining moment in my career. I realized that the corn flour in the chicken product, along with the potato flour in the cheese, and the three forms of added sugar in the salad dressing had caused a spike in Vince's blood sugar. Subsequently, his pancreas secreted insulin to divert some of the glucose from the bloodstream to the fat cells, causing the formation of triglycerides (storage fat). In these metabolic conditions, fat cells are in suppression and, therefore, incapable of both degrading triglyceride and mobilizing fatty acids. This means your fat cells are incapable of releasing fat and your body will be unable to lose fat weight.▶▶▶

After this day, I began to look for patterns: if people were consuming pre-shredded, pre-cubed, or pre-crumbled cheeses, I saw an immediate reduction in the fuel utilization of fatty acids. I also noticed another pattern. If people consumed most deli meats, they would have an abrupt decline in fat utilization. This is because most deli meats contain hidden sugar and potato flour, corn flour, or other sneaky carbohydrates such as tapioca starch. The list of uncommon terms related to unnecessary fillers is almost endless. Then I started to look at salad dressings and I realized that most salad dressings contain dextrose (sugar) and modified food starch (corn flour, which functions as a thickener), and I knew I was onto something.

As my research progressed, I wrapped up the first trial and moved into the second trial. Although my first observations about how the enzyme HSL worked first occurred in 2000, my formal instructions to avoid insidious carbohydrates in three specific categories: deli meats, salad dressings, and cheese, were not instituted until the start of the second trial. You may ask, "Why did you limit your instruction of insidious carbohydrates to just those three categories?" It's because they were staples in the regimen that I was prescribing.

It was through the observations I made during the course of the first trial and start of the second trial that I established a non-invasive technique to monitor the function of HSL, and thus accomplished my first research objective.

CHAPTER 5

The Research Continues! A Scientific Explanation for Your Weight Loss Plateau

In this chapter, you will learn that body fat weight loss plateaus can be predicted scientifically (provided that you're being guided by the most up-to-date scientific principles). Yes, you read that correctly! We *can* predict when the body begins to resist further fat loss neurologically, hormonally, and enzymatically at the cell level before it ever happens.

Much to your bewilderment, you will learn that in overweight adult female subjects, the brain will tolerate 61 to 73 percent body fat weight loss without perceiving a threat to metabolic homeostasis. In overweight adult males, the brain will tolerate 71 to 80 percent body fat weight loss without a perceived threat. This chapter will lay out exactly what the previous statements actually mean.

After matriculating into the Ph.D. program at Union Institute, I recruited a team of scientists from all over the country: field experts in human nutrition, exercise physiology, bio-physics, neuroscience, psychology, and statistics.

My dissertation was entitled "Observations of Body Fat Weight Loss with Three Different Levels of Carbohydrate Restriction."

As I touched on before, 308 overweight, non-type I diabetic, adult human subjects were divided into three human trials. The basis of all three trials was exactly the same. The subjects followed a low to moderate protein, moderate fat, high-fiber diet (half the diet came from low sugar, non-starchy vegetables) with the removal of all obvious sugars and starches from the diet. This was coupled with metabolically-controlled gentle aerobic exercise (maximizing fatty acid utilization instead of glucose). In addition, exercise was targeted for fairly light or a twelve on the Borg scale of perceived exertion for both breathing and body exertion.

See the Borg scale below:

BORG SCALE PERCEIVED EXERTION	
6	
7	VERY, VERY LIGHT
8	
9	VERY LIGHT
10	
11	FAIRLY LIGHT
12	
13	SOMEWHAT HARD
14	
15	HARD
16	
17	VERY HARD
18	
19	VERY, VERY HARD

Source: The Plourdé Institute based upon "The Borg RPE Scale" (Borg, 1998)

Subjects checked in on the phone daily (later that switched to daily text messages) and came into the laboratory once a week for body weight measurements and metabolic measurement testing. All subjects were instructed to maintain caloric neutrality. Remaining calorically neutral means that you neither have a significant calorie surplus, nor a major calorie deficit (I explain this in greater detail in chapter 7). Their prescribed calorie target was determined based on lean body mass measurements in the BOD POD. They underwent body composition testing in the BOD POD once every four weeks to determine changes in body fat weight and lean mass. Subjects were tracked for up to twelve months with the main goal of determining when and where a plateau occurred in body fat weight loss. The only difference in the three human trials was the following:

The **first group** had *no knowledge of the presence of insidious sugars and starches.*

The **second group** *had limited knowledge of the presence of insidious sugars and starches (instructions were given to avoid hidden carbohydrates in* **three categories only: deli meats, salad dressings, and cheese)**. That's because these items were staples in the daily regimen.

However, **the third group** was given **comprehensive instructions to avoid insidious sugars and starches in** *all categories of foods, fluids, and products that were ingested.*

The goal of my research was to observe the impact of insidious carbohydrates (those sugars and starches that could not be smelled, tasted, or detected) and their influence on body fat weight loss outcomes. I hypothesized that the subjects in the third trial would experience greater body fat weight loss than the subjects in the first and second groups. And that's exactly what I observed.

Using the 95 percent confidence interval, a statistical tool that predicts outcomes within a very narrow range, the following results were calculated:

Women had a 95 percent probability of losing the following percentage of their peak body fat weight:

FIRST TRIAL	SECOND TRIAL	THIRD TRIAL
46-52%	52-61%	61-73%

Men had a 95 percent probability of losing the following percentage of their peak body fat weight:

FIRST TRIAL	SECOND TRIAL	THIRD TRIAL
55-60%	65-72%	71-80%

These outcomes occurred regardless of age, and the implications of comorbidities associated with obesity were dramatically alleviated across the board.

When we combined the results for men and women among the three trials, the mean or average body fat weight loss was the following:

FIRST TRIAL	SECOND TRIAL	THIRD TRIAL
53%	63%	71%

When the statistical analysis was completed with the help of Dr. Brad Lindell, I was shocked. After a long and grueling journey, I had found what I set out to accomplish: to have a scientific framework of body fat weight loss expectations for overweight adults following the most up-to-date principles of interdisciplinary science.

Although applying these ideas may not always be easy, it is doable. The goal of this book is to **replace your pain and lead you on a path that leads to better health, joy, and self-respect**. It's often been said that you can't give someone else something you don't have for yourself. Well, I conducted this research *for you*. Let's put all these pieces together and get this problem behind you.

In order to show you how powerful the 95 percent confidence interval is in predicting when and where body fat weight loss will plateau, I'd like to share Sandy's client case study:

▶▶▶ Sandy came in for a weight loss assessment on September 6, 2012. She was fifty-seven years old, held a Doctorate in Education, and was living her best life professionally and personally. However, the little-known secret in Sandy's life was that she had struggled with a weight problem for over thirty years. If there was a diet book, she tried it. If there was a weight loss pill, she took it. If there was a new weight loss program, she would join it. All to no avail. That's when she heard about THE PLOURDE METHOD℠.

On the day of her assessment, I learned that nine years prior, at the age of forty-eight, her highest weight ever was 165 pounds, with 90 pounds of fat and 75 pounds of lean tissue. On that same day, we measured her in the BOD POD at a total weight of 153.7 pounds with 77.7 pounds of fat and 76 pounds of lean tissue. Based upon that historical data, we set forth to predict a body fat weight loss plateau using the 95 percent confidence interval.

I want to remind you that the problem that I encountered that inspired me to conduct this formal research began with Jennifer, the lady from Batavia, Illinois, who went from 139 pounds of body fat but stopped losing when she achieved approximately 70 pounds of body fat weight loss. This plateau occurred despite her near-perfect diet and exercise compliance in the program. This was an outcome that was confusing and frustrating to Jennifer and me, but it was also fascinating. I thought to myself, "Certainly Jennifer and other clients, both men and women, should be able to lose more than 50 percent of their peak body fat weight, shouldn't they?"

Based upon the analysis of Sandy's weight loss assessment and taking into consideration the 95 percent confidence interval, it was predicted that she would plateau at a level somewhere between 35.1 to 24.3 pounds of fat, or between 61 percent and 73 percent less than the peak body fat weight.

As Sandy was carefully monitored over the course of her nine-month weight loss journey, she hit a hard stop at approximately 24 pounds of fat regardless of near-perfect program compliance. It can be theorized that at this point Sandy's body was resisting further fat cell weight reduction in an effort to defend overall metabolic homeostasis. This is a fair and reasonable takeaway because the 95 percent confidence interval has held up over many years with male and female subjects regardless of their age.

Technically, her body fat loss at her plateau occurred just outside of the 95 percent confidence interval. Statistically speaking, there is a 5 percent chance that the body fat weight loss plateau occurs slightly above or below the stated range. In the case of Sandy, it was slightly above the range, which means it was even better than predicted!

When you look at her spreadsheet and graph, you will see plainly that her body fat level plateaued in the 20-to-25-pound range. She experienced mathematically linear body fat weight loss from September 6, 2012, through about July of 2013, and then body fat loss leveled off. Let me remind you, I predicted this outcome in advance. Everything that occurred was methodically mapped out during her assessment.

Sandy stated that the weekly sessions allowed her to process psychological and emotional factors that had previously set her back with unhealthy eating behaviors. These accountability sessions not only allowed her to prevent these pitfalls, but also gave her the opportunity to celebrate her successes in the program, both small and large. Through her process, she made strides not only with improved stress management, but also approached how she managed her life. The body fat weight loss outcome that she achieved had significant and positive health implications: her cholesterol levels reduced, and she experienced an increase in bone density and improved sleep patterns. Perhaps the greatest outcome was to be relieved of the constant preoccupation with unsuccessful weight loss. She had been freed from a life-long burden of thoughts focused on dieting to a new life of better health, joy, and self-respect. ▶▶▶

Scan the QR code and hear Sandy's story as she tells it herself:

The Research Continues! A Scientific Explanation for Your Weight Loss Plateau

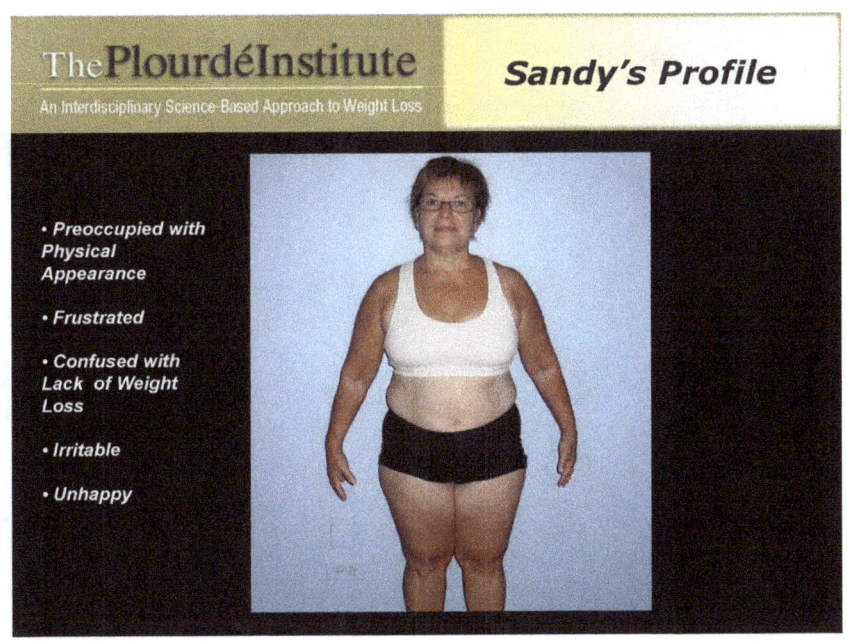

The Plourdé Institute — An Interdisciplinary Science-Based Approach to Weight Loss

Hero of the story: Sandy

- Highly Educated- Doctoral Credentials
- Highly Successful Career
- Affluent
- Happily Married
- Living a Nice Lifestyle
- Winning in Almost Every Area of Life

The Plourdé Institute — An Interdisciplinary Science-Based Approach to Weight Loss

Sandy's Profile

- Preoccupied with Physical Appearance
- Frustrated
- Confused with Lack of Weight Loss
- Irritable
- Unhappy

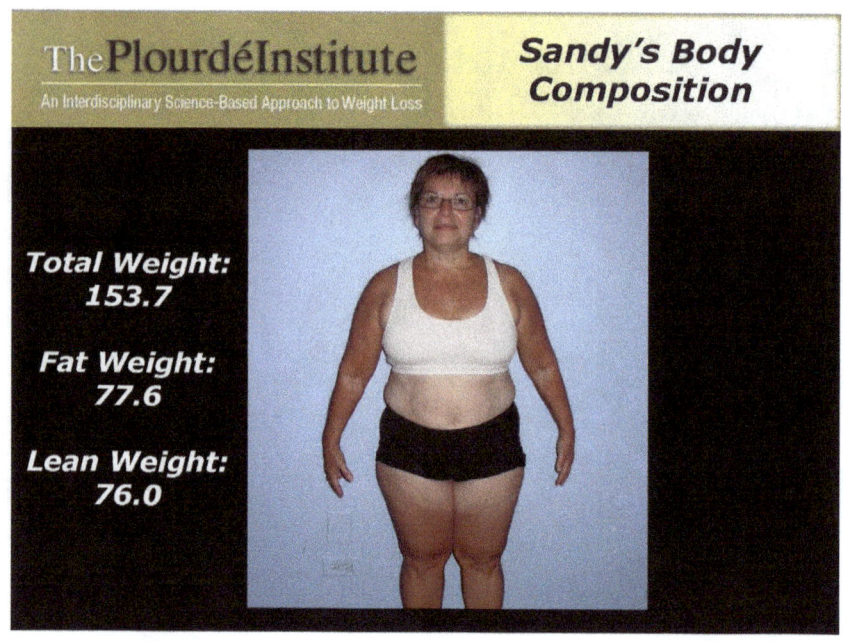

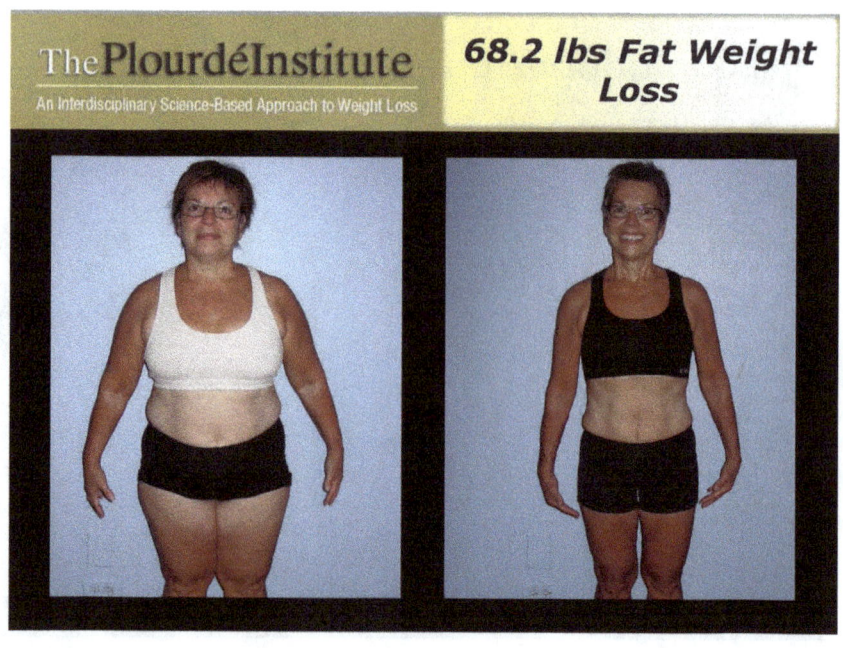

The Plourdé Institute
An Interdisciplinary Science-Based Approach to Weight Loss

Historical Evaluation of Adiposity

Name _____Sandy_____ Date _____9/6/2012_____

Condition of Adiposity	Baseline	Peak	Current	Goal - 50%	Goal - 61%	Goal - 67%	Goal - 73%
Body Fat %	25.0	54.5	50.5	36.6	30.5	27.1	23.3
Fat Weight	25.0	90.0	77.7	45.0	35.1	29.7	24.3
Lean Weight	75.0	75.0	76.0	78.0	80.0	80.0	80.0
Total Weight	100.0	165.0	153.7	123.0	115.1	109.7	104.3
Age	16	48	57	57	57	57	57
# of Adipocytes	18.9	34.0	34.0	34.0	34.0	34.0	34.0

Fat Weight Increase of _____65.0_____ lbs. = _____260.0_____ %

Type of Lipogenesis =

(Type 1) Adipocyte Hypertrophy ☐

(Type 2) Adipocyte Hyperplastic Hypertrophy (Both Types) ☐

Fat Weight Reduction Goal: 32.7 lbs = 42.1 %
                             42.6 lbs = 54.8 %
                             48.0 lbs = 61.8 %
                             53.4 lbs = 68.7 %

Estimated Range of Reduction Phase = _6-9_ months

Copyright © 2023 David Plourdé, Ph.D.

Credit: The Plourdé Institute

34   Solving the Weight Loss Puzzle

BODY COMPOSITION PROGRESS CHART

CLIENT NAME: SANDY   GOAL FAT WEIGHT: 27.0

DATE	TOTAL WEIGHT	FAT WEIGHT	LEAN WEIGHT	FAT LOSS	% FAT LOSS	TOTAL FAT LOSS
9/6/2003	165.0	90.0	75.0			
9/6/2012	153.7	77.6	76.0	12.34	-13.7%	12.34
10/3/2012	144.2	66.5	77.7	11.10	-14.3%	23.43
10/31/2012	135.7	57.3	78.4	9.30	-14.0%	32.73
11/28/2012	129.6	49.8	79.7	7.43	-13.0%	40.16
1/2/2013	123.4	43.3	80.1	6.51	-13.1%	46.67
1/30/2013	117.6	36.7	80.9	6.58	-15.2%	53.25
3/6/2013	114.8	33.4	81.4	3.34	-9.1%	56.58
4/3/2013	110.6	28.2	82.4	5.18	-15.5%	61.77
5/1/2013	109.9	26.5	83.4	1.70	-6.0%	63.46
5/29/2013	109.0	24.4	84.6	2.14	-8.1%	65.60
7/2/2013	110.7	26.0	84.7	-1.61	+6.6%	63.99
7/31/2013	109.6	23.4	86.2	2.62	-10.1%	66.60
9/4/2013	108.5	21.8	86.6	1.55	-6.6%	68.15
10/2/2013	108.9	22.3	86.6	-0.46	+2.1%	67.68
10/30/2013	110.2	23.5	86.7	-1.21	+5.4%	66.48
12/11/2013	109.7	23.0	86.7	0.49	-2.1%	66.97
1/16/2014	112.1	25.5	86.6	-2.53	+11.0%	64.44
2/12/2014	111.1	24.7	86.3	0.80	-3.1%	65.24
4/1/2014	113.7	27.2	86.5	-2.43	+9.8%	62.81
5/6/2014	114.5	27.9	86.5	-0.77	+2.8%	62.04
6/10/2014	115.4	28.8	86.6	-0.86	+3.1%	61.18
7/9/2014	116.3	29.9	86.4	-1.05	+3.7%	60.12
8/6/2014	114.4	27.9	86.5	1.99	-6.7%	62.11
9/3/2014	113.9	27.4	86.5	0.48	-1.7%	62.59
10/1/2014	112.0	25.5	86.5	1.88	-6.9%	64.47
11/5/2014	112.7	26.1	86.5	-0.63	+2.5%	63.84
12/10/2014	113.0	26.4	86.6	-0.26	+1.0%	63.58

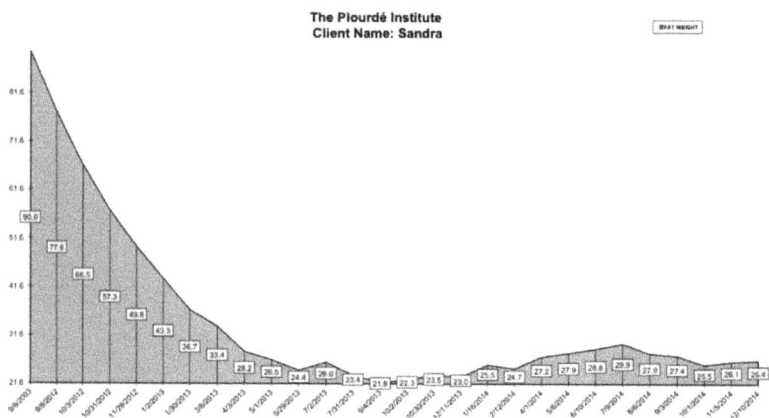

The Plourdé Institute
Client Name: Sandra

DATE

CHAPTER 6

If Your Fat Cells Could Talk, They'd Say: "ABSOLUTELY NOT!"

Let me explain: physiologically speaking, your inability to lose body fat is the result of an enzyme suppression within the human fat cell. The enzyme Hormone-Sensitive Lipase (HSL), which we talked about previously, is a special mechanism that regulates individual fat cell weight. When this enzyme is in a state of suppression, it renders the fat cell incapable of degrading triglyceride (the chemical name for storage fat), subsequently making it practically impossible for the release of what are called fatty acids (just a fancy way of saying fat).

The other important point I want to add is that fat cells are not static: they don't sit still. At any given moment, fat cell weight is either going up or down. This means that if your fat cells are in a state of suppression, they are predisposed for the creation of new triglyceride. In other words, fat cell weight can only go up in a state of suppression. **Therefore, having control of this enzyme mechanism is a fundamental necessity for effective fat weight loss.**

36   Solving the Weight Loss Puzzle

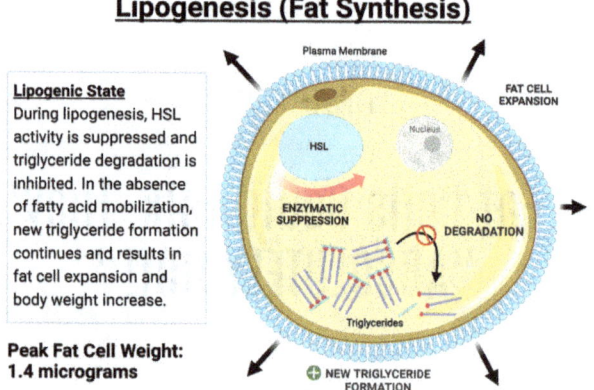

Credit: Created in BioRender. Plourde, D., Plourde, B. (2024) BioRender.com/b68u802

This chapter will carefully explain how THE PLOURDE METHOD℠ re-activates the enzyme in the fat cells so that they swiftly say "YES" to the **degradation** of fat and "YES" to the CONTINUOUS **mobilization of fatty acids**.

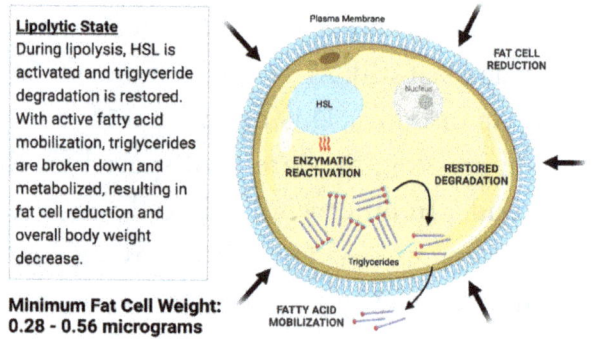

Credit: Created in BioRender. Plourde, D., Plourde, B. (2024) BioRender.com/d16y439

I cannot overstate the importance of the previous statement. *The reason why successful weight loss has eluded you is because you've never had control of this enzyme mechanism.* It borders on the impossible for a person to have substantial fat loss when the fat cells are in a state of suppression. The content in this chapter will be a defining moment for you. As you contemplate your own frustrating weight loss efforts in the past, I think you'll find that this idea is a concrete explanation for why your efforts were not effective. And let me add, you cannot exercise your way out of this suppression state. This chapter will outline how to have greater control of this mechanism.

Scan this QR code to watch my video about this exact concept:

It's a well-established fact that low carbohydrate diets are the most effective for weight loss. But why? The answer lies inside of your fat cells. When a person ingests sugar or starch in a manner that is either obvious or insidious, fat cells are incapable of breaking fat and releasing it for multiple days for **each instance.**

This means that when you're following a weight loss regimen, and you unknowingly ingest sugar in a manner that you can't smell, taste, or detect, there is a period of time when fat cells can only get larger, resulting in body fat increases. This is one of the main reasons why weight loss can be such a demoralizing endeavor. In many of the attempts you've made to lose weight in the past, you have accidentally tripped into suppression, but the problem is you can't see it. You can't detect it. It's invisible unless you're in a laboratory setting. I've been sharing these observations exclusively with my private clients for decades, but now want to make them available to you in this book.

Here you will find Diagram I of the human fat cell and Diagram II the human fat cell with HSL in a state of suppression:

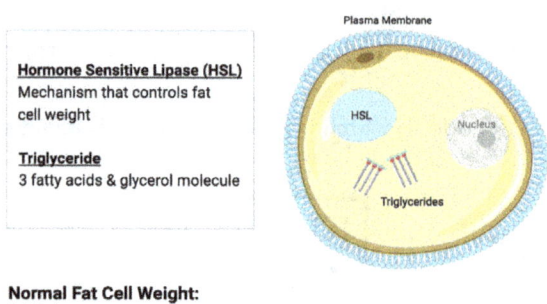

Credit: Created in BioRender. Plourde, D., Plourde, B. (2024) BioRender.com/m65f625.

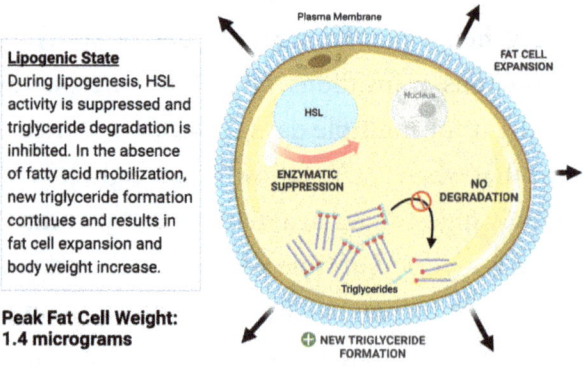

Credit: Created in BioRender. Plourde, D., Plourde, B. (2024) BioRender.com/b68u802

So, I know we have discussed elements of the fat cell previously, but I'd like to pull it all together. That being said, some of the information may be redundant, but I want to make sure you understand it.

Every cell in the human body has a cell membrane. It's called a phospholipid. The lipid refers to fat. This means that the outer shell of every cell is made of fat, but it's not the kind of fat your body can use for fuel. It's more of a structure—like your bones.

Every cell has a nucleus. The nucleus functions like the brain of the cell. Typically, the nucleus is located in the center, but *not* in your fat cells. Fat cells are different. The nucleus in the fat cell is located all the way to the side.

The inner space of the cell is called the cytoplasm. This is where your fat cells manufacture fat. The chemical name for fat is triglyceride. Triglycerides are composed of two components: first is the *tri* part—triglycerides are composed of three fatty acids. These three fatty acids are held together by the second component of the triglyceride: glycerol. Glycerol is an alcohol molecule.

Every fat cell has an enzyme mechanism called—you guessed it—**Hormone-Sensitive Lipase (HSL)**. This enzyme controls the individual weight of every fat cell. This is where the problem lies: in over thirty-three years of laboratory experience, every person I've conducted a science-based weight loss assessment for has come into our laboratory and their fat cells were in a state of suppression. You might ask, *"How do you know this?"* I've measured the metabolism of thousands of overweight human subjects utilizing an FDA-approved metabolic measurement cart. Among these thousands of documented cases, fat was minimally available as a fuel source, thus the body defaulted to the utilization of glucose. This is an irrefutable fact.

40   Solving the Weight Loss Puzzle

> **TRUTH: Cellular respiration yields the metabolic byproducts of heat, water, and carbon dioxide gas.**

The heat from cellular respiration yields your resting body temperature of approximately 98.6 degrees. When a person dies, cellular respiration ceases and the body literally becomes cold in a matter of minutes.

The second byproduct of cellular respiration is water. The water comes out of your cells and eventually through your skin in the form of sweat. When the air hits the skin, the water evaporates and it cools the body temperature back down to normal.

The third byproduct, carbon dioxide gas, exits the cell, enters the blood, and circulates. It then diffuses from the blood, through the lungs, and ultimately out through the exhaled breath.

So, why did I go to the trouble to explain this process to you? Because when fat cells are in suppression, fatty acids are unavailable as a fuel source and, as I mentioned earlier, the body defaults to the utilization of glucose. Under these metabolic conditions, the cells give off a much higher level of carbon dioxide gas.

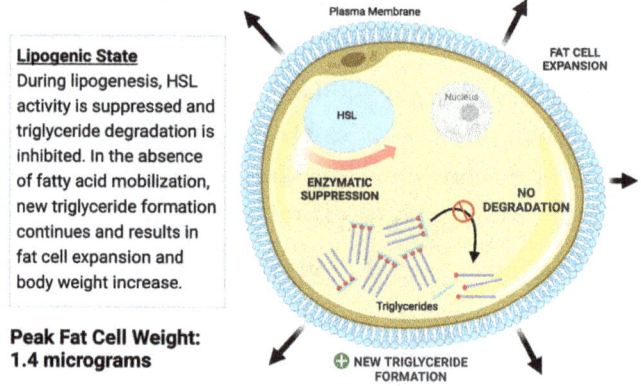

Credit: Created in BioRender. Plourde, D., Plourde, B. (2024) BioRender.com/b68u802

Conversely, when HSL is re-activated and fat cells mobilize fat continuously, the fatty acids become available as the primary fuel source in cellular work, yielding markedly less carbon dioxide gas.

In application, if your fat cells are in suppression, HSL shuts down any chance of your fat cells from breaking the triglyceride into pieces, subsequently blocking any mobilization of fatty acids. Moreover, fat cells in a state of suppression can only manufacture new triglycerides, which means that when you're in suppression, fat cells can only get larger and heavier.

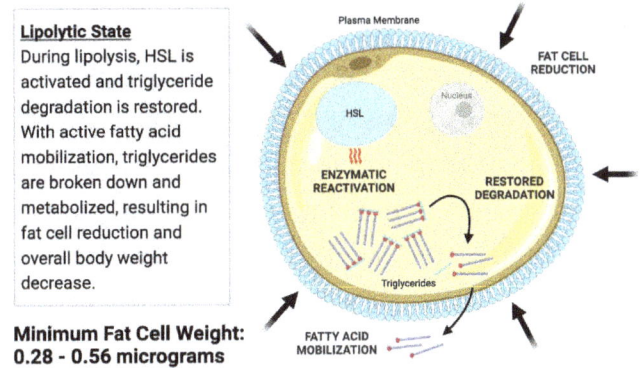

Created in BioRender. Plourde, D., Plourde, B. (2024)
BioRender.com/d16y439

FACT: Your body fat weight is simply the weight of all your fat cells.

When fat cells are in suppression, body fat can only go up! And you cannot exercise yourself out of the state of suppression. This may seem like you're doomed, but actually, the opposite is true.

Throughout my career, I've observed the chemical quality of the things that people ingest in foods, fluids, and products AND their relationship to the function of HSL and the implications on body fat weight loss and body fat weight gain.

What came out of my formal research was that the essence of the meal plan *was* effective in producing substantial fat loss. However, greater fat loss occurred as the subjects in the second and third trials were made progressively more aware of the presence of hidden sugars and starches (and how to avoid them) and its influence on HSL.

At the onboarding of each subject, the scientific METHOD was thoroughly explained. As the individuals were able to grasp how it worked, I noticed that people inevitably felt hopeful about their likelihood of success. This then translated to a higher level of motivation and greater levels of compliance. Consistent compliance produced predictable body fat weight loss that perpetuated increased hope, and the cycle continued. There was nothing accidental about it.

Getting back to the research, I want to mention something: when you look at the differences in body fat weight loss outcomes among the three trials, you might be wondering how there was such a significant difference in what total fat weight loss could be. It has to do with how *precisely reactive* HSL is.

When someone ingests sugar or starch, blood sugar elevates. The pancreas subsequently releases insulin—a hormone that reduces blood sugar. Insulin helps divert excess blood glucose to the fat cells where it is converted to triglyceride or storage fat. As I mentioned before, the differences between body fat weight loss in the first trial and the third trial were quite significant, and that has to do with how ridiculously sensitive HSL is to even the most minute secretions of insulin.

You see, when insulin is secreted, it signals HSL into suppression, only allowing fat synthesis and simultaneously preventing fat mobilization. In application, that means that *even hidden sugars and starches* will trigger a suppression that lasts for multiple days in each instance. That means that if a person ingests a hidden carbohydrate more than once per week, there can be no substantial body fat weight loss for that week. This is why the weight loss process can be so confusing and frustrating at times. People unknowingly step into suppression in all directions, but they can't see it and they can't detect it because it's invisible.

Let's examine a real-life case study:

▶▶▶ Chuck, a fifty-nine-year-old senior sales executive, demonstrated this aspect of our weight loss program. He came to the Institute on August 5, 2016, for a weight loss assessment. The results revealed that Chuck's highest body weight was 362 pounds, at which point he maintained 203 pounds of fat and 159 pounds of lean tissue. When we placed him in our human performance laboratory and measured his metabolic conditions, we observed that fat was minimally available as a fuel source, and that his body was running predominantly on glucose to drive cellular respiration. This was evidence of the suppression of HSL.

Chuck entered the program and implemented the meal plan immediately. At his next appointment, cellular respiration had shifted from almost entirely glucose utilization to almost entirely fatty acid utilization. Simply stated, his body switched from using sugar to fat as its primary fuel source . . . in less than one week! Chuck fully complied with THE PLOURDE METHOD℠ and enjoyed full control of his fat cells for an entire year, resulting in mathematically linear body fat weight loss as outlined in the reports in the pages ahead.

This change in metabolic conditions and the control of the fat cells was depicted in his body composition test results. From August 5, 2016, his body fat weight reduced at nearly 12 percent per month (every month) through October 2017. His body fat weight went from 203 pounds at the peak to just over 30 pounds at the plateau, representing an 81.3 percent body fat weight loss. In the coming pages, you will see his spreadsheet depicting these results, along with his Historical Evaluation of Adiposity (this is a term that I coined in the 1990s that reflects changes in body fat over the course of a person's lifetime).

As previously mentioned with Sandy's case study, the 95 percent confidence interval predicts that body fat weight loss will plateau, with a 95 percent probability, somewhere between 71 and 80 percent. However, let me remind you, there is a 5 percent chance that the plateau occurs just before or just after the interval. In Chuck's case, body fat weight loss occurred just above the interval. Keep in mind that the 95 percent confidence interval applies to THE PLOURDE METHOD℠ only and not to other weight loss approaches. ▶▶▶

If Your Fat Cells Could Talk, They'd Say: "ABSOLUTELY NOT!"

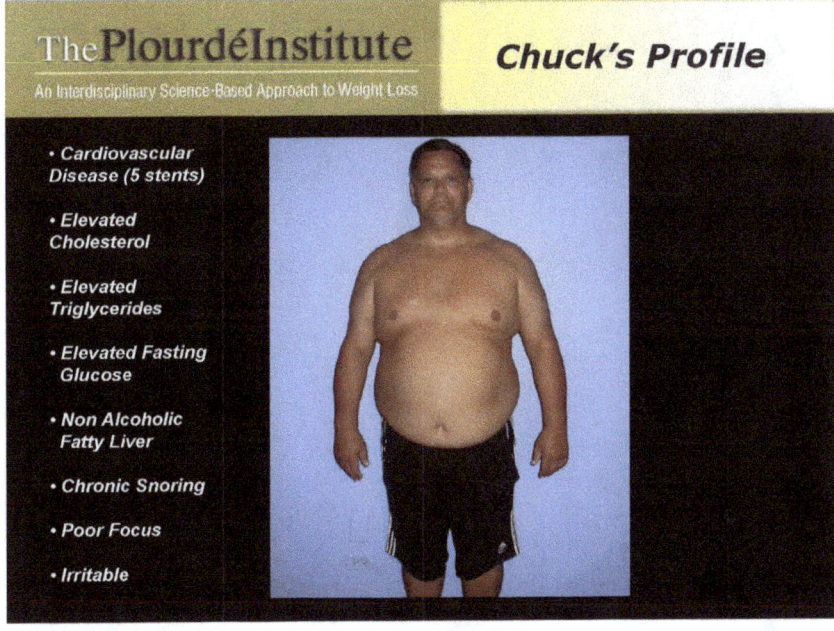

The Plourdé Institute — An Interdisciplinary Science-Based Approach to Weight Loss

Hero of the story: Chuck

- Successful Business Leader
- Affluent
- Married with Two Awesome Kids
- Living a Nice Lifestyle
- Winning in Almost Every Area of Life

The Plourdé Institute — An Interdisciplinary Science-Based Approach to Weight Loss

Chuck's Profile

- Cardiovascular Disease (5 stents)
- Elevated Cholesterol
- Elevated Triglycerides
- Elevated Fasting Glucose
- Non Alcoholic Fatty Liver
- Chronic Snoring
- Poor Focus
- Irritable

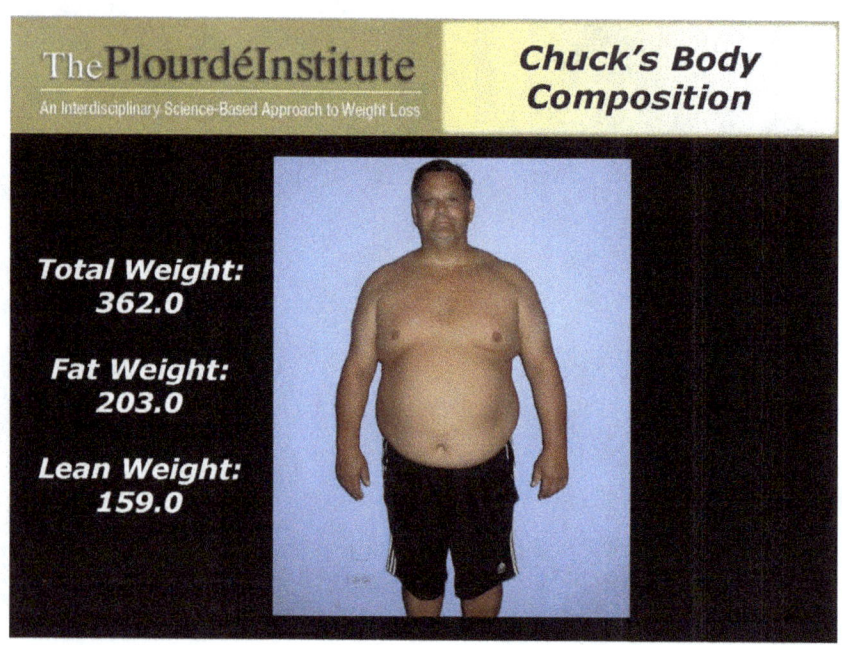

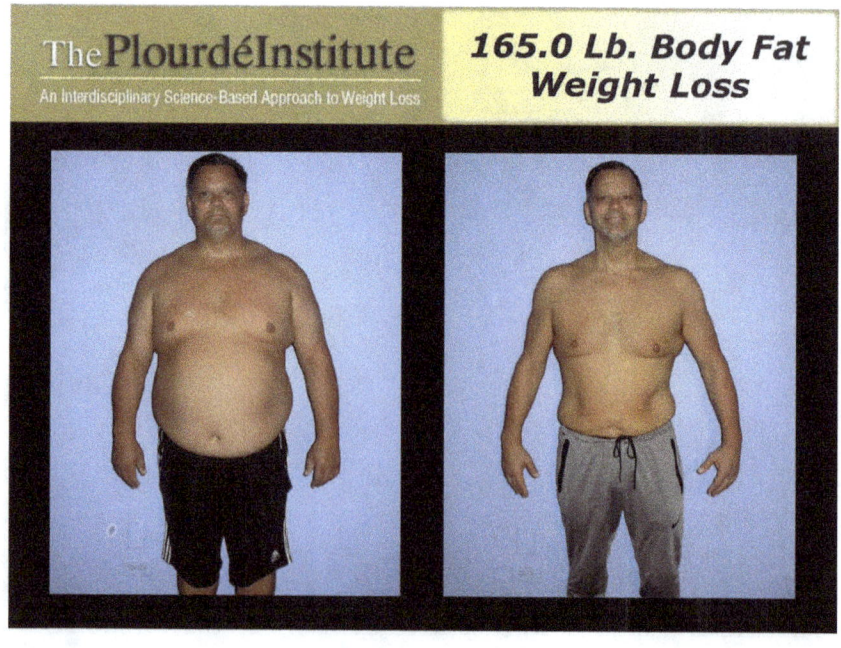

If Your Fat Cells Could Talk, They'd Say: "ABSOLUTELY NOT!" 47

The Plourdé Institute
An Interdisciplinary Science-Based Approach to Weight Loss

Historical Evaluation of Adiposity

Name _____Chuck_____   Date __8/5/2016__

Condition of Adipocity	Baseline	Peak	Current	Goal - 50%	Goal - 60%	Goal - 71%	Goal - 75%	Goal - 80%
Body Fat %	6.0	56.1	48.8	38.6	33.1	26.1	23.3	19.5
Fat Weight	9.9	203.0	151.7	101.5	81.2	58.9	50.8	40.6
Lean Weight	155.1	159.0	159.0	161.7	164.4	167.1	167.1	167.1
Total Weight	165.0	362.0	310.7	263.2	245.6	226.0	217.9	207.7
Age	22	54	56	56	56	56	56	56
# of Adipocytes	7.5	76.7	76.7	76.7	76.7	76.7	76.7	76.7

Fat Weight Increase of __193.1__ lbs. = __1950.5__ %

Type of Lipogenesis =

(Type 1) Adipocyte Hypertrophy ☐

(Type 2) Adipocyte Hyperplastic Hypertrophy (Both Types) ☐

Fat Weight Reduction Goal: 50.2 lbs = 33.1 %
                            70.5 lbs = 46.5 %
                            92.8 lbs = 61.2 %
                           101.0 lbs = 66.5 %
                           111.1 lbs = 73.2 %

Estimated Range of Reduction Phase = __7-9__ months

Copyright © 2023 David Plourdé, Ph.D.

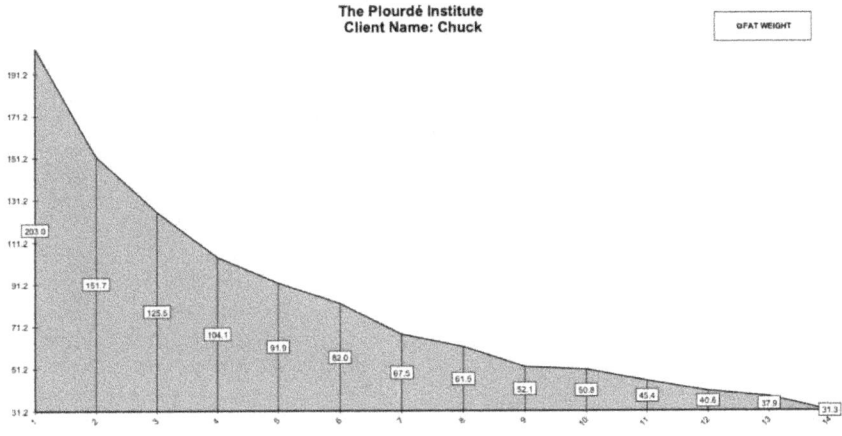

The Plourdé Institute
Client Name: Chuck

DATE

The Plourdé Institute
An Interdisciplinary Science-Based Approach to Weight Loss

BODY COMPOSITION PROGRESS CHART

CLIENT NAME: CHUCK B   **GOAL FAT WEIGHT: 28.4**

DATE	TOTAL WEIGHT	FAT WEIGHT	LEAN WEIGHT	FAT LOSS	% FAT LOSS	TOTAL FAT LOSS
1/5/2015	362.0	203.0	159.0			
8/5/2016	310.7	151.7	159.0	51.27	-25.3%	51.27
9/10/2016	286.0	125.5	160.6	26.29	-17.3%	77.56
10/22/2016	264.7	104.1	160.6	21.38	-17.0%	98.94
11/19/2016	253.0	91.9	161.1	12.20	-11.7%	111.14
12/17/2016	244.6	82.0	162.5	9.85	-10.7%	120.99
1/28/2017	232.7	67.5	165.2	14.55	-17.7%	135.55
3/4/2017	227.0	61.5	165.5	5.93	-8.8%	141.48
4/8/2017	218.8	52.1	166.7	9.48	-15.4%	150.96
6/3/2017	218.1	50.8	167.3	1.29	-2.5%	152.25
7/14/2017	215.4	45.4	170.0	5.38	-10.6%	157.63
8/19/2017	210.7	40.6	170.1	4.81	-10.6%	162.44
9/16/2017	208.2	37.9	170.3	2.65	-6.5%	165.09
10/14/2017	204.7	31.3	173.4	6.68	-17.6%	171.76

Scan the QR code to hear Chuck's amazing story:

CHAPTER 7

The Most Crucial Puzzle Piece: Your Meal Plan

Of all of the pieces that comprise your weight loss puzzle, this one is THE most important. If you get this wrong, nothing is going to go right. I need your full attention.

In this chapter, you will learn what **to** eat and drink and what **not to** eat and drink. You will also learn about ideal meal frequency, timing between meals, and your specific calorie target. Having said that, as a reminder, the principles that I've laid out in this chapter are not the full breadth of intellectual property and trade secrets that I've accumulated throughout my career, but it does include the heart of the overall METHOD, which will allow you to accomplish greater than 50 percent body fat weight loss from your peak fat weight.

The Meal Plan

Let's dive in! This meal plan, simply stated, is a low to moderate protein, moderate fat, high-fiber diet (half the diet should come from non-sugary, non-starchy vegetables) with the removal of both obvious and insidious sugars and starches from the diet.

In the pages ahead, you will find gender-specific guidance for what you should eat and drink. Instructions on how to access a more complete list of Plourdé metabolically-approved brands and products will be included in the Personal Invitation chapter.

What TO Eat and Drink

Females:

- ☐ 2 to 4 ounces of fresh proteins at breakfast, lunch, and dinner. This can come from eggs, chicken breast or thighs, fresh seafood, pork, and limited beef (to prevent constipation).

- ☐ 1 to 1.5 tablespoons of pure fat with breakfast, lunch, and dinner. This source of fat could come from butter, olive oil, avocado oil, avocado, or nut butters (without sugar, of course). You may also use Marie's brand Ranch, Caesar, or Creamy Italian Garlic salad dressing (search on the Marie's website for where those are available, and please note that only these three Marie's dressings meet our criteria). This fat source should be above and beyond the butter or oil you cook with because some of that fat source burns off in the pan in the cooking process. This detail will encourage consistent and productive bowel movements. Understand that it's not recommended that you double up on your fat sources, because this will result in calorie surpluses exceeding your calorie target. More will be mentioned about your calorie target later.

- ☐ Half of your diet should come from non-sugary, non-starchy vegetables, preferably raw or lightly cooked: broccoli with some stem, cauliflower, celery, and cucumbers are great choices.

*I would like to mention that for certain people, raw vegetables can cause difficulty with digestion. If this is you, lightly cook your vegetables—keeping in mind that cucumbers are soft by nature and don't require being cooked. If, historically, you have problems digesting certain vegetables, such as broccoli, it can be replaced with another vegetable, such as lightly cooked asparagus. Apply common sense here. If you have any known food allergies, please avoid those foods and select an alternative that your body agrees with.

- ☐ Drink mostly unflavored water. Black coffee and LaCroix sparkling water are also acceptable in moderation. LaCroix, specifically, is allowed because the essence is composed of an aromatic fruit oil, not sugar or juice (which are included in many other similar products on the market). A rare or occasional diet soda such as Diet Coke, Coke Zero, 7-Up Zero Sugar, or Sprite Zero Sugar is allowed.

A Word About Alcohol For Females

Alcohol can be allowed in a successful weight loss journey, but you need to keep these specific factors in mind:

The calorie density of alcohol is similar to that of fat or oil. Alcohol contains seven calories per gram and oil or fat contains nine calories per gram. Therefore, if a person is not mindful of the portions of alcohol they consume, she may experience imperceptible calorie spikes that stop successful weight loss in its tracks. To be clear, weight loss is more likely to be successful without alcohol being ingested. If you do consume alcohol, I suggest that it be one or two nights a week at a quantity of one to two drinks per night.

Unfortunately, it's important to avoid beer, wine, sangria, most cocktails, and any sweetened alcoholic beverages. Tequila is not on plan because it has a high sugar content. Whiskey, bourbon, and scotch have a greater alcohol content and caloric density, and therefore can slow the weight loss process down. The best options, metabolically speaking, are vodka or gin.

Males:

- ☐ 4 to 8 ounces of fresh proteins at breakfast, lunch, and dinner. This can come from eggs, chicken breast, chicken thighs, fresh seafood, pork, and limited beef (to prevent constipation).

- ☐ 1.5 to 2 tablespoons of pure fat with breakfast, lunch, and dinner. This source of fat could come from butter, olive oil, avocado oil, avocado, or nut butters (without sugar, of course). You may also use Marie's brand Ranch, Caesar, or Creamy Italian Garlic salad dressing (search on the Marie's website for where those are available, and please note that only these three Marie's dressings meet our criteria). This fat source should be above and beyond the butter or oil you cook with because some of that fat source burns off in the pan in the cooking process. This detail will encourage consistent and productive bowel movements. Understand that it's not recommended that you double up on your fat sources, because this will result in calorie surpluses exceeding your calorie target. More will be mentioned about your calorie target later.

- ☐ Half of your diet should come from non-sugary, non-starchy vegetables, preferably in a raw or lightly cooked state: broccoli with some stem, cauliflower, celery, and cucumbers are great choices.

*I would like to mention that for certain people, raw vegetables can cause difficulty with digestion. If this is you, lightly cook your vegetables—keeping in mind that cucumbers are soft by nature and don't require being cooked. If, historically, you have problems digesting certain vegetables, such as broccoli, it can be replaced with another vegetable, such as lightly cooked asparagus. Apply common sense here. If you have any known food allergies, please avoid those foods and select an alternative that your body agrees with.

- ☐ Drink mostly unflavored water. Black coffee and LaCroix sparkling water are also acceptable in moderation. LaCroix, specifically, is allowed because the essence is composed of an aromatic fruit oil, not sugar or juice (which are included in many other similar products on the market). A rare or occasional diet soda such as Diet Coke, Coke Zero, 7-Up Zero Sugar, or Sprite Zero Sugar is allowed.

A Word About Alcohol For Males

Alcohol can be allowed in a successful weight loss journey, but you need to keep these specific factors in mind:

The calorie density of alcohol is similar to that of fat or oil. Alcohol contains seven calories per gram and oil or fat contains nine calories per gram. Therefore, if a person is not mindful of the portions of alcohol they consume, he may experience imperceptible calorie spikes that stop successful weight loss in its tracks. To be clear, weight loss is more likely to be successful without alcohol being ingested. If you do consume alcohol, I suggest that it be one or two nights a week at a quantity of one to two drinks per night.

Unfortunately, it's important to avoid beer, wine, sangria, most cocktails, and any sweetened alcoholic beverages. Tequila is not on plan because it has a high sugar content Whiskey, bourbon, and scotch have a greater alcohol content and caloric density, and therefore can slow the weight loss process down. The best options, metabolically speaking, are vodka or gin.

The following is a quick reference guide for the effective avoidance of insidious sugars and insidious starches. This is NOT a list of bad foods. As I mentioned earlier, all foods are good. Rather, the question is whether the item is metabolically optimum for you or not. So, the real question is: does this food trigger a suppression of the HSL enzyme? This list will help you to avoid both the obvious as well as the sneaky carbohydrates that you might not have thought of. Clearly, this is not an all-inclusive list, but I hope you find it to be helpful!

What NOT to Eat and Drink

The Plourdé Method ®

<u>What Not To Eat</u>

Bread	Corn	Iced tea
Crackers	Peas	Coffee with flavored syrups
Pretzels	Beans	Citrus fruits
Croutons	Green beans	Lemon on meats or vegetables
Cookies	Beets	Sugar or vinegar containing
Potato chips	Peppers	marinades
Corn chips	Hot peppers or giardiniera	Pre-shredded cheese
Tortilla chips	Onions (raw and cooked)	Pre-cubed cheese
Cheese puffs	Radish	Pre-crumbled cheese
Tortilla wraps	Garlic (raw and cooked)	Reduced-fat cheese
Pita bread	Garlic powder	Any Cheese with Natamycin
Pita chips	Onion powder	
Waffles	Leeks	Meat with Sugar in it:
Pancakes	Zucchini, okra and squash	Bacon
Donuts	Olives	Sausage
Bagels	Pickles	Ham
Brownies	Avoid fruit in general (however	
French fries	after initial weight loss, you may	Highly Salted Meat:
Hash browns	include limited amounts of	Prosciutto
Onion rings	berries and apples)	Salami
Scones	Rice	Roast Beef
Pudding	Pasta	Gyro Meat
Bread pudding	Potato	Pepperoni
Cake	Couscous	Corned beef
Cheesecake	Cereal	Most deli meat
Pie	Oatmeal	Other pre-packaged meat (fresh
Pizza	Granola	meat located in the meat
Pastry	Popcorn	department of your grocery store
Croissants	Salted nuts	is on plan as long as it does not
Biscuits	All Candy	have added ingredients)
Breaded foods	All Desserts sweetened with	
Tomatoes	sugar	
Tomato sauce	Meal replacement bars	Chewing gum
Tomato paste	Protein bars	Breath strips
Salsa	"Keto" products	Breath mints
Ketchup	Fruit and vegetable juices	Flavored floss picks
Hot sauce	Ice cream	Mouthwash
Steak sauce	Yogurt	Regular soda
Mustard	Milk, soy or most nut-based milks	
Vinegar	(Some brands of Heavy Whipping	
Gravy	Cream are on plan)	
Au jus	Whipped cream sweetened with	
Barbecue, soy, teriyaki, and	sugar	
peanut sauce	Water with fruit in it	
Table salt	Fruit flavored water (except	
Pre-made soup and broth	LaCroix)	
Carrots	Tea	

Credit: The Plourdé Institute

How To Eat

Before I go any further, I would like to clear up a misnomer: the idea of predetermined general calorie intake at 1,200 calories per day for women and 2,000 calories for men needs to be thrown out, and here is why. I'd like to share a personal story. As I mentioned earlier, I was a former Illinois state champion competitive powerlifter. My highest bench press was 525 pounds. I could squat over 700 pounds and run the forty-yard dash in 4.5 seconds. I always saw myself as the former athlete who could eat and drink pretty much anything and not gain weight. That all changed when I hit forty years old. I started gaining weight, and it's fair to say that the weight loss doctor shouldn't be overweight, right? The truth is that I was upset and really uncomfortable with this uptick. Let me preface what I'm about to say by sharing with you: I had not conducted a resting metabolic rate measurement on myself up until this point. My own dietary habits were predicated upon my perceptions only. And it turns out, this was a huge blind spot for me.

Let me pause to give you a brief explanation of what the resting metabolic rate measurement is: it is the amount of energy your body expends in a resting state over a twenty-four-hour period. In other words, if you laid down on a couch and did absolutely nothing for an entire day, how much energy would your body expend?

I assumed that my resting metabolic rate would be somewhere around 2,200 calories to 2,400 calories given my body build. What I'm about to share with you was a profound embarrassment for me. When I *actually* measured my resting metabolic rate in the laboratory, it was only 1,670 calories. My perception had been so alarmingly inaccurate! I was off by 530 to 730 calories, and this is what I do for a living. So, if *I* got it wrong (and I got it WAY wrong), how much more likely is a non-science person to overestimate their resting metabolic rate and subsequently their calorie target? The answer is: very likely. And it's probably one of the reasons why you've been unsuccessful in your weight loss efforts.

FACT: Your calorie target should be correlated with the weight of your lean tissue, not your total weight.

This can most accurately be determined by body composition testing in a laboratory. However, I have developed a Calorie Target Calculator which I am making available to you. This framework is based on my experience working with thousands of overweight subjects in a clinical setting. Let me forewarn you: your bathroom scale's bioelectrical impedance measurement is only a gross estimation and may be inaccurate. **Instructions on how to access the Plourdé Calorie Target Calculator will be included in the Personal Invitation chapter.**

Once an accurate body composition measurement has been conducted for you, your calorie target may be determined. To make this easy to understand, I have created a chart that correlates lean body mass to the appropriate calorie targets for small, medium, and large framed females and males, respectively.

Just to be perfectly clear, for those of you who have a lean mass somewhere in between the ten-pound increments, you can round down or round up. If you are halfway between (eighty-five pounds, ninety-five pounds, etc.), the calorie target will be 850, 950, etc.

Female	Approximate Lean Mass	Suggested Calorie Target
Small Body Frame	80 to 90 pounds	800 to 900 calories
Average Body Frame	100 pounds	1,000 calories
Large Body Frame	110 to 130 pounds	1,100 to 1,300 calories

Male	Approximate Lean Mass	Suggested Calorie Target
Small Body Frame	130 to 140 pounds	1,300 to 1,400 calories
Average Body Frame	150 pounds	1,500 calories
Large Body Frame	160 to 200 pounds	1,600 to 2,000 calories

There are exceptions that don't fall into this structure. Let me give you a few examples. The smallest framed adult female I have ever measured had seventy-one pounds of lean tissue. I mentioned earlier that I had worked with the Buffalo Bills and I have also worked with the Chicago Bears in guiding them in using the BOD POD effectively. According to Rusty Jones, the strength coach for the Buffalo Bill and the Chicago Bears, Hall of Fame linebacker Brian Urlacher had a lean mass of over 238 pounds.

My point here is that there is a massive disparity in lean mass among human beings, which leaves the opportunity for major errors in determining your calorie target.

As you can see, if people institute the general calorie recommendation from the dietetics model, they will experience calorie surpluses every twenty-four hours. Let's assume for a moment that a person is replicating a low to moderate protein, moderate fat, high fiber diet absent of obvious sugars and starches. None of that would matter. **The body has the capacity to convert proteins and fats and anything else that you consume to a triglyceride: in the liver, this process is called lipogenesis. In application, in the presence of a calorie surplus, even without insulin secretion or HSL suppression, fat cells grow and body fat weight increases.**

Let me say it one more time: if you replicate a calorie surplus—knowingly or unknowingly—and everything you consumed was entirely free of both obvious and insidious sugars and starches, **fat cell weight and body fat weight still goes up.**

Have you ever asked yourself the question, "As careful as I am with my diet, how could I not be losing weight?" This could very well be your answer. Unfortunately, to know your calorie target, you need to look objectively and accurately at your body composition. Frustratingly, your perceptions, your bathroom mirror, your scale, and the general guidelines are failing you. The essence of what I'm trying to convey here is that **you *must* maintain caloric neutrality**.

What Is Caloric Neutrality?

Remaining calorically neutral means that you neither have a significant calorie surplus, nor a major calorie deficit. As we will later discuss, when a metabolically-controlled exercise prescription is followed, muscle fibers exclusively utilize mobilized fatty acids from the fat cells sparing muscle glycogen. Therefore, the METHOD couples the mobilization of fatty acids with the uptake and utilization of fatty acids.

Your calorie intake should be correlated to your resting metabolic rate and matched to your lean body mass and not your total weight. To be more clear, calories ingested above the resting metabolic rate that are not used up (utilized in cellular respiration) will be converted to triglycerides in your fat cells, *even if the fat cells are not in suppression*, resulting in body fat weight gain.

> **Warning: adding your expended exercise calories back onto your daily calorie target is a common mistake, and it may be a contributing factor to your unsuccessful weight loss efforts.**

This may be hard for you to accept, but in a later chapter, you will learn that *Metabolically-Controlled Exercise* (as part of THE PLOURDE METHOD[SM]) will pinpoint the utilization of exclusively mobilized fatty acids and not any substantial amount of sugar in your muscle contractions. The brain will tolerate this fuel utilization without any perceived threat or spike in hunger or sugar cravings because of the nature of the incredible fuel efficiency that fatty acids provide.

Please be mindful of these things and track your calories.

How Often Should I Eat?

The short answer is: eat every two and a half hours whether you're hungry or not. This may seem strange to you; however, eating on this interval will prevent the feeding centers of the brain from even activating. This part of the brain regulates hunger and satiety and is located right behind your eyes in the center of your head. See diagram of the feeding centers:

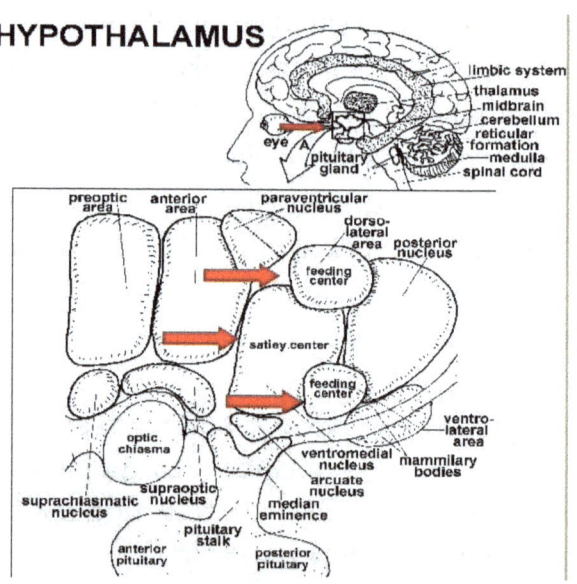

Source: (Kapit, Macey and Meisami, 1987)

What am I saying? This means that you will be, in effect, NEVER HUNGRY. You may have a hard time believing this, but it works like clockwork. While no lab test can prove this, the absence of hunger has been a benefit of the METHOD reported by the thousands of people that I've guided through the process. You will notice that this common experience is mentioned firsthand in many, if not all, of the client success story videos that are available throughout this book and on our websites.

In application, start with eating breakfast, and then two and a half hours later you will eat a mini meal (some examples include: raw, unsalted almonds; raw, unsalted peanuts; or cucumbers or celery if you suffer from diverticulitis). Then, two and a half hours later you will eat lunch. Two and a half hours after that, you will have another mini-meal. Two and a half hours later, you eat dinner. You get the picture.

There is no eating after dinner. There is no night eating. I typically suggest dinner to be between 5:00 and 6:30 p.m., if possible. Obviously, there will be exceptions to this principle for those of you who have unconventional work hours.

This goes back to the idea of caloric neutrality. If you ingest a level of calories above the resting metabolic rate, and these calories ARE NOT UTILIZED THROUGH EXERCISE, the excess calories will be inter-converted to a triglyceride, regardless of whether it was a protein, fat, or carbohydrate. This means that the body will synthesize or manufacture new fat in your fat cells, EVEN IF THEY ARE NOT IN SUPPRESSION.

In addition, if you have difficulty determining fullness, preset your portions according to your calorie targets, and do not exceed them.

To reiterate, I want you to eat every two and a half hours whether you're hungry or not. Here are some examples of calorie targets and subsequent meal plans to give you an idea of where we are going. I will provide instructions on how to access a more complete set of options for calorie target and meal plan information in the Personal Invitation chapter.

1000 Calorie Meal Plan Example (100 pound lean mass)

#1 Option

*Breakfast — Calories
2 eggs + 3 Tbs. Egg White Omelet (165)
1 tsp Butter (34)
1 Cup Broccoli (30)
2 Cup Spinach (14)
½ oz. Provolone (50) (293)

*Mini Meal
10 Almonds (70)

*Lunch
4 oz. Roasted Chicken Breast (188)
1 Cup Cauliflower (25)
2 tsp Marie's Ranch Dressing (60) (273)

*Mini Meal
1 Cup Cucumber (15)
½ Tbs. Peanut Butter (50) (65)

*Dinner
3 oz. Sirloin Steak (175)
1 Cup Cauliflower (25)
1 Cup Broccoli (30)
2 tsp. Marie's Ranch Dressing (60) (290)
Total (991)

#2 Option

*Breakfast — Calories
2 eggs + 3 Tbs. Egg White Scramble (165)
1 Cup Mushroom (16)
1 Cup Broccoli (30)
½ oz. American Cheese (50)
1 tsp Butter (34) (307)

*Mini Meal
1 Cup Cucumber (15)
½ Tbs. Peanut Butter (50) (65)

*Lunch
3 oz. Extra Lean Ground Burger (95% lean) (117)
½ oz. American Cheese (50)
2 Cups Cauliflower (50)
2 tsp Marie's Ranch Dressing (60) (277)

*Mini Meal
1.5 Tbs. Sunflower Seeds (81)

*Dinner
3 oz. Salmon (177)
1 tsp Olive Oil (40)
1 Cup Broccoli (30)
1 Cup Cauliflower (25) (271)
Total (1001)

#3 Option

*Breakfast — Calories
2 eggs + 3 Tbs. Egg White Omelet (165)
1 Cup Asparagus (27)
1 Cup Broccoli (30)
½ oz. American Cheese (50) (272)

*Mini Meal
10 Almonds (70)

*Lunch
3 oz. Chicken Breast (140)
1 Cup Cucumbers (15)
1 Cup Broccoli (30)
1 Tbs. Marie's Ranch Dressing (90) (275)

*Mini Meal
1 Cup Celery (14)
1 tsp. Peanut Butter (64) (78)

*Dinner
3 oz. Pork Tenderloin (122)
2 tsp Olive Oil (80)
1 Cup Cauliflower (25)
1 Cup Celery (14)
½ Tbs. Marie's Ranch Dressing (45) (286)
Total (981)

#4 Option

*Breakfast — Calories
2 eggs + 3 Tbs. Egg White Scramble (165)
1 tsp. Butter (34)
½ oz. Fresh Mozzarella (45)
1 Cup Asparagus (27)
1 Cup Cauliflower (25) (296)

*Mini Meal
1 Cup Cucumber (15)
½ Tbs. Peanut Butter (50) (65)

*Lunch
2 Lettuce Wraps (2)
4 oz. Applegate Farms Turkey (100)
½ oz. American Cheese (50)
1 Cup Broccoli (30)
1 Cup Cucumber (15)
1 Tbs. Marie's Caesar Dressing (85) (282)

*Mini Meal
10 Almonds (70)

*Dinner
4 oz. Grilled Tilapia (112)
2 Cups Cauliflower (50)
½ tsp. Butter (17)
½ Tbs. Marie's Ranch Dressing (45)
½ oz. Parmesan Cheese (65) (289)
Total (1007)

Credit: The Plourdé Institute

The Most Crucial Puzzle Piece: Your Meal Plan

1500 Calorie Meal Plan Example (150 pound lean mass)

#1 Option

*Breakfast — Calories
2 eggs + 6 Tbs. Egg White Omelet (190)
1 tsp. Butter (34)
2 Cups Broccoli (60)
1 oz. Cheddar Cheese (114)
(398)

*Mini Meal
20 pcs. Almonds (140)

*Lunch
4 oz. Chicken Breast (187)
2 tsp. Olive Oil (80)
1 Cup Broccoli (30)
1 Cup Cauliflower (25)
1 Tbs. Marie's Ranch Dressing (90)
(412)

*Mini Meal
20 pcs. Almonds (140)

*Dinner
4 oz. Sirloin Steak (234)
2 tsp. Butter (68)
1 Cup Cauliflower (25)
1 Cup Broccoli (30)
½ Tbs. Marie's Caesar Dressing (43)
(400)
Total
(1490)

#2 Option

*Breakfast — Calories
2 eggs + 6 Tbs. Egg White Omelet (190)
1 tsp. Butter (34)
1 Cup Broccoli (30)
1 Cup Cauliflower (25)
1 ½ oz. Swiss Cheese (159)
(438)

*Mini Meal
20 pcs. Almonds (140)

*Lunch
3 oz. (85/15) Ground Beef (180)
2 tsp. Olive Oil (80)
1 Cup Broccoli (30)
1 Cup Cauliflower (25)
1 Tbs. Marie's Italian Garlic Dressing (90)
(405)

*Mini Meal
2 ½ Tbs. Unsalted Sunflower Seeds (131)

*Dinner
6 oz. Cod (168)
1 Tbs. Butter (102)
1 Cup Broccoli (30)
1 Cup Cauliflower (25)
2 tsp. Marie's Ranch Dressing (60)
(385)
Total
(1499)

#3 Option

*Breakfast — Calories
2 eggs + 6 Tbs. Egg White Omelet (190)
1 tsp. Butter (34)
2 Cups Broccoli (60)
1 oz. Cheddar Cheese (114)
(398)

*Mini Meal
20 pcs. Almonds (140)

*Lunch
6 oz. Applegate Oven Roasted Turkey Breast (150)
1 oz. Pepper jack Cheese (100)
1 tsp. Olive Oil (40)
2 Cup Cauliflower (50)
2 tsp. Marie's Caesar Dressing (56)
(396)

*Mini Meal
20 pcs. Almonds (140)

*Dinner
6 oz. Lobster Tail (168)
1 Tbs. Butter (102)
1 Cup Cauliflower (25)
1 Cup Broccoli (30)
1 Tbs. Marie's Italian Garlic (90)
(415)
Total
(1489)

#4 Option

*Breakfast — Calories
2 eggs + 6 Tbs. Egg White Omelet (190)
1 tsp. Butter (34)
2 Cups Broccoli (60)
1 oz. Colby Cheese (110)
(394)

*Mini Meal
20 pcs. Almonds (140)

*Lunch
6 oz. Shrimp (180)
2 tsp. Olive Oil (80)
2 Cup Cauliflower (50)
1 Tbs. Marie's Ranch Dressing (90)
(400)

*Mini Meal
2 ½ Tbs. Unsalted Sunflower Seeds (131)

*Dinner
4 oz. Bison Filet (190)
1 tsp. Butter (34)
1 Cup Cauliflower (25)
1 Cups Broccoli (30)
2 tsp. Olive Oil (80)
2 tsp. Marie's Ranch Dressing (60)
(419)
Total
(1484)

Credit: The Plourdé Institute

To help you further maintain caloric neutrality, I've included a calorie reference chart to help you keep track of your daily calorie intake:

The Plourde Institute
Calorie Tracker

EGGS			**DAIRY**		
Egg Whites	2 Tbs	16.5	Heavy Whipping Cream	1 tsp	17
3 T = 1 Whole Egg	3 Tbs	25		.5 Tbs	25
Eggs	1	70		1 Tbs	50
Hard-boiled Eggs	1	70		2 Tbs	100
			Butter	1 tsp	34
CHEESE				.5 Tbs	51
Cheddar	.5 oz	57		1 Tbs	102
	1 oz	114		2 Tbs	204
	2 oz	228	Sour Cream	1 tsp	10
Swiss	.5 oz	53.5		.5 Tbs	15
	1 oz	107		1 Tbs	30
	2 oz	214		2 Tbs	60
Feta	.5 oz	33.5	Mayo	1 tsp	30
	1 oz	67		.5 Tbs	45
	2 oz	134		1 Tbs	90
Mozzarella	.5 oz	45		2 Tbs	180
	1 oz	90	Cream Cheese	1 Tbs	50
	2 oz	180		2 Tbs	100
Pepperjack	.5 oz	50		3 Tbs	150
	1 oz	100	Cottage Cheese	1 Tbs	14
	2 oz	200		2 Tbs	28
Parmesan	.5 oz	65		3 Tbs	42
	1 oz	130	**NUTS**		
	2 oz	260	Almonds	10 pcs	70
Goat Cheese	.5 oz	35		15 pcs	105
	1 oz	70		20 pcs	140
	2 oz	140	Pinenuts	1 Tbs	48
American	.5 oz	50		2 Tbs	96
	1 oz	100	Sunflower Seeds	1 Tbs	54
	2 oz	200		2 Tbs	108
Colby	.5 oz	55	Pumpkin Seeds	1 Tbs	80
	1 oz	110		2 Tbs	160
	2 oz	220	**ALCOHOL**		
Provolone	.5 oz	49	Vodka(Tito's)	1.5 oz	70
	1 oz	98		3 oz	140
	2 oz	196	Gin(Hendrick's)	1.5 oz	108
Muenster	.5 oz	50		3 oz	216
	1 oz	100	Whiskey(Jack Daniel's)	1.5 oz	98
	2 oz	200		3 oz	196
			Red Wine		
			Pinot Noir	5 oz	120
			Merlot/Cab.	5 oz	122
			White Wine		
			Chardonnay	5 oz	123
			Pinot Grigio	5 oz	120

Credit: The Plourdé Institute

The Plourde Institute
Calorie Tracker

Vegetables

Item	Serving	Calories	Item	Serving	Calories
Broccoli	1/2 cup- 1.5 oz	15	Artichoke Hearts	1/2 cup- 3oz	52
	1 cup- 3 oz	30		1 cup- 5.9oz	104
	2 cups- 6 oz	60		2 cups-11.8oz	208
Cauliflower	1/2 cup- 2 oz	12.5	Zucchini	1/2 cup-2.2 oz	10
	1 cup- 4 oz	25		1 cup-4.3 oz	21
	2 cups- 8 oz	50		2 cups-8.6 oz	42
Celery	1/2 cup-2oz	7			
	1 cup-4oz	14			
	2 cups-8oz	28			
Asparagus	1/2 cup-2.4 oz	13.5			
	1 cup- 4.8 oz	27			
	2 cups- 9.6 oz	54			
Cucumber	1/2 cup- 1.8 oz	7.5			
	1 cup- 3.6 oz	15			
	2 cups- 7.2 oz	30	**Dressing**		
Avocado	1/4 of whole	80	Clara's		
	1/2 of whole	160	Ranch	1 tsp	20
	Whole	320		.5 Tbs	30
Mushrooms	1/2 cup- 1.25 oz	8		1 Tbs	60
	1 cup- 2.5 oz	16		2 Tbs	120
	2 cups- 5 oz	32	Gorgonzola	1 tsp	20
Spinach	1/2 cup- 0.55 oz	3.5		.5 Tbs	30
	1 cup- 1.1 oz	7		1 Tbs	60
	2 cups- 2.2 oz	14		2 Tbs	120
Romaine	1/2 cup- 0.85 oz	4			
	1 cup- 1.7 oz	8			
	2 cups- 3.4 oz	16			
Kale	1/2 cup- 1.2 oz	16.5			
	1 cup-2.4 oz	33	Marie's		
	2 cups-4.8 oz	66	Ranch	1 tsp	30
Arugula	1/2 cup- 0.35 oz	3		.5 Tbs	45
	1 cup- 0.7 oz	6		1 Tbs	90
	2 cups- 1.4 oz	12		2 Tbs	180
Brussel Sprouts	1/2 cup- 1.5 oz	19	Caesar	1 tsp	28
	1 cup-3 oz	38		.5 Tbs	42.5
	2 cups-6 oz	76		1 Tbs	85
Bok Choy	1/2 cup-1.25 oz	4.5		2 Tbs	170
	1 cup-2.5 oz	9	Italian Garlic	1 tsp	30
	2 cups-5 oz	18		.5 Tbs	45
Butter Lettuce	1/2 cup- 1 oz	3.5		1 Tbs	90
	1 cup- 2 oz	7		2 Tbs	180
	2 cups- 4 oz	14			
Mustard Greens	1/2 cup- 1 oz	7.5			
	1 cup- 2 oz	15			
	2 cups- 4 oz	30			

Credit: The Plourdé Institute

The Plourde Institute
Calorie Tracker

MEATS			FISH		
Chicken Breast	2 oz	94	Salmon	2 oz	118
	4 oz	188		4 oz	236
	6 oz	282		6 oz	354
Ground Chicken	2 oz	50	Tilapia	2 oz	56
	4 oz	100		4 oz	112
	6 oz	150		6 oz	168
Turkey Breast	2 oz	76	Mahi Mahi	2 oz	48
	4 oz	152		4 oz	96
	6 oz	228		6 oz	144
Ground Turkey	2 oz	60	Cod	2 oz	56
99% Lean	4 oz	120		4 oz	112
	6 oz	180		6 oz	168
Deli Turkey	2 oz- 2 slices	50	Halibut	2 oz	106
Applegate/Dietz & Watson	4 oz- 4 slices	100		4 oz	212
	6 oz- 6 slices	150		6 oz	318
Ground Beef	2 oz	120	Lobster	2 oz	56
85% lean	4 oz	240		4 oz	112
	6 oz	360		6 oz	168
Beef Tenderloin	3 oz	90	Shrimp	2 oz	60
	6 oz	180		4 oz	120
	8 oz	240		6 oz	180
Beef Round	2 oz	130	Crab(lump)	2 oz	48
	4 oz	260		4 oz	96
	6 oz	390		6 oz	144
Ground Bison	2 oz	100	Scallops	2 oz	63
	4 oz	200		4 oz	126
	6 oz	300		6 oz	189
Bison Steak	2 oz	82	Yellowfin Tuna	2 oz	74
	4 oz	164		4 oz	148
	6 oz	246		6 oz	222
Pork Tenderloin	2 oz	82	Striped Bass	2 oz	54
	4 oz	164		4 oz	108
	6 oz	246		6 oz	162
Pork Chop	2 oz	110	Grouper	2 oz	52
	4 oz	220		4 oz	104
	6 oz	330		6 oz	156
Lamb	2 oz	168	Mussels(meat)	2 oz	98
	4 oz	336		4 oz	196
	6 oz	504		6 oz	294
Veal (ground)	2 oz	100	Oysters(meat)	2 oz	46
	4 oz	200		4 oz	92
	6 oz	300		6 oz	138
Cornish Game Hen	2 oz	110	Clams	2 oz	50
	4 oz	220		4 oz	100
	6 oz	330		6 oz	150

Credit: The Plourdé Institute

The Plourde Institute
Calorie Tracker

MEATS			FISH		
Sirloin Steak	2 oz	138	Swordfish	2 oz	82
	4 oz	276		4 oz	164
	6 oz	414		6 oz	294
Strip Steak	2 oz	66	Chilean Sea Bass	2 oz	106
	4 oz	132		4 oz	212
	6 oz	198		6 oz	318
CONDIMENTS			Walleye	2 oz	68
Olive Oil	1 tsp	40		4 oz	136
	1 Tbs	120		6 oz	204
Peanut Butter	1 tsp	32	Orange Roughy	2 oz	45
	1 Tbs	95		4 oz	90
Tamari (low sodium)	1 tsp	5		6 oz	135
	1 Tbs	15	Barramundi	2 oz	62
Sesame Oil	1 tsp	43		4 oz	124
	1 Tbs	130		6 oz	186
Coconut Oil	1 tsp	40			
	1 Tbs	120			
Swanson's Chicken Stock	1/2 Cup	10			
	1 Cup	20			

Credit: The Plourdé Institute

Subsection: Seven Factors to Prevent Constipation in Your Weight Loss Journey

The following content is invaluable information regarding a common potential pitfall in weight loss that you probably didn't see coming. Warning: the following subject may be perceived as embarrassing and difficult to discuss, but it is an absolute necessity for effective weight loss. I'll also preface this following section by making clear that I am not a gastroenterologist.

Believe it or not, your bowel movements can have a significant impact on your weight loss journey. Let me explain: for every day that your evacuations (my way of saying bowel movements) are less than stellar, your body weight may be clouded by somewhere between 1 and 2 pounds of un-evacuated material per day, and it's accumulative. Unfortunately, constipation is very common in weight loss for many reasons. This annoying issue confuses, frustrates, and, in some cases, demoralizes people because they perceive they're not losing weight when, in fact, they're literally full of you know what.

To help you to prevent this problem in your own weight loss journey, let me share with you **seven leading causes of constipation in weight loss:**

1. **You're not eating enough vegetables. Half of your diet should come from vegetables.** More specifically, raw or lightly cooked vegetables like broccoli with some stem, cauliflower with some stem, and celery (celery is recommended almost always in a raw form). If you have difficulty digesting these vegetables, you can replace them with others, such as cucumbers, asparagus, spinach, brussel sprouts, or any of

the vegetables listed on the Calorie Tracker. The common denominator among these vegetables is that they do not contain sugar or starches, but provide a lot of bulk, water, and some fiber, all of which help your body to form larger, softer stools. In application, this translates to approximately two cups of vegetables at each main meal (six cups total per day). If you're anything like my wife, she can't eat the primary vegetables mentioned earlier. She consumes her vegetables in a lightly cooked manner. Everybody is different. So please pay attention to how your body responds to this aspect of the program and adjust it accordingly.

2. **You're not drinking enough water.** The best indicator of your hydration status is your urine output. Urine should be produced in a relatively large quantity and be slightly yellow to clear. Keep in mind that the weather can play a significant role in how much water you require. If, for example, you're experiencing high heat and humidity, you'll perspire more, and thus need much more water. Conversely, in cold and dry climates, you'll experience the opposite and may need less water.

"The U.S. National Academies of Sciences, Engineering, and Medicine determined that an adequate daily fluid intake is:

- About 15.5 cups (approximately 125 ounces) of fluids a day for men
- About 11.5 cups (approximately 91 ounces) of fluids a day for women" (Mayo Clinic Staff, 2022)

Furthermore, for those of you who suffer from congestive heart failure, blood pressure, or kidney issues, seek specific guidance from your medical doctor. The important thing here is to avoid the dangers of dehydration (not enough water) and water intoxication (too much water). We will talk about this in the next subsection.

3. **You're eating too much cheese. Limit cheese intake.** Keep cheese at somewhere between zero to two ounces daily. Too much cheese slows peristalsis (the muscle contractions of the digestive tract) and causes constipation. Let me also say that you should avoid cheese as a mini meal for the same reason. However, for some people, cheese accelerates peristalsis. For example, those who suffer from lactose intolerance can have a spastic reaction to cheese and other dairy products, causing loose stools. I'm not suggesting that a lactose-intolerant person should eat lots of cheese to encourage frequent bowel movements, so please apply common sense here. If your evacuations are slow, make sure you're asking yourself about your cheese intake and adjust it accordingly.

4. **You may need more fiber. Take supplemental fiber.** I recommend the consumption of whole, raw flaxseed as a "go to" fiber source. Generally, I recommend that fiber be taken after dinner. With flaxseed, the recommended dose is somewhere between four and six tablespoons. You may say to yourself, "That seems like a lot." Well, it is, but it definitely works.

Instructions on how to take flaxseed are included here:

The Plourdé Institute
An Interdisciplinary Science-Based Approach to Weight Loss

Nutrition Supplementation

Supplement	Dosage	Additional Protocol
Whole Raw Flax Seed	6 Tablespoons	1 x Daily • After Dinner • Immediately after chase with water.
		Swallow Whole in Small Amounts - Do Not Chew
		Chased With Large Amount of water
		Allow <u>at least 2 hour separation</u> between Vitamins /Medications and taking Flax Seed
		Drink Plenty of Water when taking flax. Inadequate water intake with flax could create choking hazard.
		Flax Seeds should be taken with <u>flat water</u>

Copyright © 2023 David Plourdé, Ph.D.

***The exception to this guideline would be if you have **diverticulitis**. This is a condition where the formation of small pockets occur on the intestinal lining. Small seeds and food particles can get caught leading to inflammation, abdominal pain, constipation, and even infection. If untreated, it may require a surgical intervention. It's important that you pay attention to your body's response to supplemental fiber. Please be mindful of this and reach out to your physician if you're having any prolonged bowel issues. If it bothers you, stop. If it doesn't, go ahead and consume.

If you don't know if you suffer from diverticulitis or have a propensity for this condition, ask your family members if they have a history with it. If there is any family history, opt for a different fiber source. Instead of the flaxseed, I would suggest taking psyllium fiber after dinner. You can take Sugar Free Metamucil®, which contains psyllium; however, there are other products on the market that have no other ingredient except psyllium husk that you can choose instead. The label suggests taking one to two heaping teaspoons with food, starting with one time per day and increasing to twice per day if well tolerated.

Instructions for how to take psyllium are included here:

The Plourdé Institute

An Interdisciplinary Science-Based Approach to Weight Loss

Fiber Supplementation

Supplement	Dosage	Additional Protocol
Sugar Free Artificially Flavored Orange Flavor Metamucil or Pure Psyllium	1-2 Heaping Teaspoons mixed with flat Water	1 x Daily • Just Before Bed
		Allow at least 2 hour separation between Vitamins /Medications and taking Psyllium

Copyright © 2023 David Plourdé, Ph.D.

5. **You're not eating enough fat. Consume one to two tablespoons of pure fat with every main meal.** Ingesting fat stimulates the production of bile salt in the liver. Bile salt travels through the bile duct and lands in the gallbladder. The gallbladder disperses bile salt into the small intestine when you eat fat through a valve called the sphincter. If you consume no fat, you get no bile. If you consume excessive amounts of fat, you'll get excessive amounts of bile. When bile salt hits the small intestine, it stimulates peristalsis.

   If you've had your gallbladder removed, you don't have a slow, steady release of bile—you have a continuous flow of bile from the liver to the small bowel because there's no gallbladder to store it. That's why when you eat a lot of fat at one time, you may have a spastic reaction and have loose stools. The point here is to be sure to have a source of pure fat with every meal: butter, olive oil, avocado oil, avocado, peanut butter (as long as you don't have an allergy), Marie's brand Ranch salad dressing, Marie's Creamy Italian Garlic, or Marie's Caesar (these are soybean oil-based salad dressings). Generally speaking, I recommend that you do not count the fat that you are cooking with, because some oil/butter will burn off in the pan. Adequate fat with breakfast, lunch, and dinner ensures consistency in peristalsis and the formation of healthy bowel movements. So, if you notice your evacuations are slow, ask yourself the question, "Am I getting enough fat with my main meals?" If not, be sure to adjust accordingly.

6. **You're eating too much protein. Protein intake should be low to moderate.** For women, I recommend two to four ounces of protein with your main meals. For men, I recommend four to six ounces of protein with the main meals.

If you consume too much protein, you'll be susceptible to constipation. This can be confusing and demoralizing in your weight loss process. Trust me on this.

7. **You're eating too much beef. Limit your beef intake**. My experience with people is that if they consume beef too frequently, it will constipate them. This is true especially for women. Please be mindful of your beef consumption. I suggest you keep beef intake to no more than once or twice per week tops. Keep in mind that in restaurant situations, a steak or a burger may be the safest option metabolically speaking (to avoid suppression of HSL). Don't fret about that. All you can do is your best.

If you are suffering from prolonged constipation, if you are straining to the point that it's painful, or if you are bleeding, or if you have abdominal pain, you need to see your physician. Chronic constipation needs to be taken very seriously. Therefore, keep these principles where you can see them regularly as a reminder of what the keys are to having consistently medium to large soft stools, and healthy bowel function. If you've undergone a bowel resection or have a colostomy bag, these principles may not be appropriate for you. People who have suffered ulcerative colitis need to pay careful attention, as well. You'll need to seek advice from your gastroenterologist in these circumstances.

Here is a Seven Factors quick reference guide:

The Plourdé Institute
An Interdisciplinary Science-Based Approach to Weight Loss

Seven Factors to Prevent Constipation

1. Consume 2 cups of CORE vegetables three times daily with meals. Vegetables that qualify as core are those that contain significant amounts of bulk, fiber and water. Therefore, emphasize broccoli, cauliflower and/or celery on a daily basis. Other vegetables classified as peripheral are also appropriate, but not necessarily from the core. They can also be consumed *in addition* to core vegetable intake.

2. Consume ample amounts of water. Urine production is the best indicator of your state of hydration. Urine production should be medium to large and clear to slightly yellow.

3. Limit cheese intake. Significant cheese consumption will constipate anyone. Limit cheese intake to 1 ounce - 1 to 2 times daily or less.

4. Take supplemental fiber. The most common recommended supplemental fiber at Plourdé is flax seed. The therapeutic dose is 6 tablespoons nightly. Flax seed must be swallowed whole. If you chew it, you'll absorb the fat calories from the oil of the flaxseed. Sugar-free Metamucil (plant fiber known as psyllium) may also be taken as a source of supplemental fiber. This would be recommended if the subject suffers from diverticulitis or diverticulosis. Small particles can cause stomachache and may interrupt peristalsis completely.

5. Consume an adequate source of fat with each meal. This would equate to 1 tablespoon per meal. Best recommendations for sources of fat would include butter, olive oil and or soy bean oil. Cheese would not fall into this category because it slows peristalsis.

6. Limit protein portions to 2-4oz per meal for women and 4-6oz per meal for men.

7. Limit beef consumption to no more than once per week.

www.theplourdeinstitute.com
901 Warrenville Road, Suite 110, Lisle, Illinois, 60532   630.769.0776

Subsection: Avoid the Pitfall of Salt Spikes and Water Retention

Another common pitfall in weight loss that my clients have experienced over the years is an overnight water retention leading to an unexplained weight gain that can range from 2 to 5 pounds, and sometimes more in certain cases. This can occur as the result of an unforeseen salt spike from things like soy sauce, Buffalo sauce, brined meats, or even having too much on-plan deli meat. Other salty foods such as olives, cured meats, or what I've coined "mystery meats" (because you never know what's really in them—like hot dogs, bratwurst, bacon, sausage, etc.) can also lead to these salt spikes. Even many traditional Thanksgiving turkeys are prepped with an injected brine of saline (salt) solution and dextrose (sugar) before they arrive at the store.

I'd like to take a moment to explain the nature of a salt spike. Physiologically speaking, there are three classifications for sodium levels in your bloodstream. "**Hypertonic**" means you have a high blood sodium level. "**Isotonic**" means you have an ideal sodium level. "**Hypotonic**" means that you have a low level of sodium in the bloodstream. You may be wondering why the body responds so sensitively resulting in these 2 to 5 pound overnight water weight gains. Well, here's the reason. The concentration and ratio of blood sodium and blood potassium plays directly into your heart rhythm. The body constantly monitors the level of what are called electrolytes because it's so important to the body's metabolic homeostasis or stability.

In a *hypertonic* state, blood sodium increases dramatically above the level of potassium. In these circumstances, the hypothalamus directs the pituitary gland and the pituitary gland directs the kidneys through the release of antidiuretic hormone. As the name indicates, it's the opposite of a diuretic, which causes the body to urinate less. The fluids that would normally be excreted through the urinary system are recirculated back into the blood supply to dilute the sodium levels. The point I want to make here is that for the body to correct from a hypertonic state to an isotonic state, or normal levels of sodium, it may require an accumulative water retention of anywhere from one to five pounds, depending on the severity of the increases in sodium concentration in the bloodstream. This can occur in literally less than twenty-four hours.

Once the ratio of sodium and potassium has been normalized, the body will drain off the excess fluid with increased urine output. You need to know that this correction could take anywhere from two to four days, and if you don't understand this, you'll be vulnerable to feeling utterly confused, frustrated, and perhaps even demoralized. And do I even need to say that these are the moments in a weight loss journey that people often quit because they have no idea what's happening?

Let's move on to talk about a *hypo*tonic or low blood sodium level. I'll explain this through the following scenario. A person is running the Chicago Marathon and, in this instance, the ambient temperature is in the mid-nineties with high humidity. The person is sweating profusely—so much so that you can see streaks of salt on their clothing. Here is where the problem comes in. The person over hydrates with water not fortified with electrolytes: sodium, potassium, calcium, and magnesium. As a result, blood sodium levels drop quickly and the water coming into the body doesn't replenish these levels. Physiologically, the body may strangely direct increased urine output draining off fluid to raise the concentration of sodium. Do you see where this is going? Sodium and potassium levels can fall so dangerously low that there's not enough electrolyte to maintain electrical conductivity in the bloodstream to produce a heart rhythm. In which case, the heart stops beating, causing death. This rare but very dangerous condition is called "water intoxication." Inevitably, you will hear in the news every so often of a person dying during a marathon from "water intoxication."

So, you can see from this example and this explanation that the body tirelessly monitors and works to maintain appropriate electrolyte levels, and it's the reason why if you ingest unforeseen high sodium foods, that it results in such a dramatic overnight water weight gain. Do not be discouraged by this, but rather pay attention to what's happening and adjust your approach.

As we wrap up this chapter, let me demonstrate the power of the Plourdé meal plan.

▶▶▶ I'd like to introduce you to client case study, Jim. At the time he came to me, he was fifty-five years old and was a significant shareholder and chairman of a bank. Jim was in the business of buying and selling banks. Needless to say, he was extraordinarily successful. He was also highly educated, holding an MBA from the prestigious Kellogg School of Management in Evanston, Illinois.

I met Jim in February 2009, when I was a guest speaker at a charitable organization that he was a member of. He approached me after my speech and asked for my business card, so I gave it to him. He quickly looked at it and realized that his bank was only a few blocks from the Institute. At that moment he looked up and said, "Okay, God, I get the message."

Jim promptly scheduled an appointment and arrived at the Institute on March 6, 2009, for an assessment. At that time, Jim suffered from arthritis in his knee, snoring, obstructive sleep apnea, and borderline type II diabetes. He was headed in a disastrous direction. Regardless of how financially successful Jim was, and no matter how happy he was in his marriage to Cathy, he was preoccupied with a profound unhappiness with his appearance, low energy, and the overall status of his health.

The results of his assessment indicated that he weighed 246.6 pounds with 166.5 pounds of lean tissue and 80.1 pounds of body fat. This was the highest Jim's body fat had ever been in his lifetime.

He began the program immediately. He followed his prescribed meal plan, and the results changed his life forever. As you will see from his spreadsheet, his body fat weight went from 80.1 pounds to 6 pounds. This was an approximate 90 percent body fat weight loss, and he has maintained this outcome for over fifteen years. In addition, he gained approximately 6 pounds of muscle. Today, at the age of seventy, Jim has less body fat than when he was seventeen years old as a competitive swimmer at Fenwick High School in Oak Park, Illinois. Here, again, is a case where the body fat weight loss plateau was outside of the 95 percent confidence interval and better than we anticipated. ▶▶▶

See Jim's spreadsheet and Historical Evaluation of Adiposity in the coming pages:

80   Solving the Weight Loss Puzzle

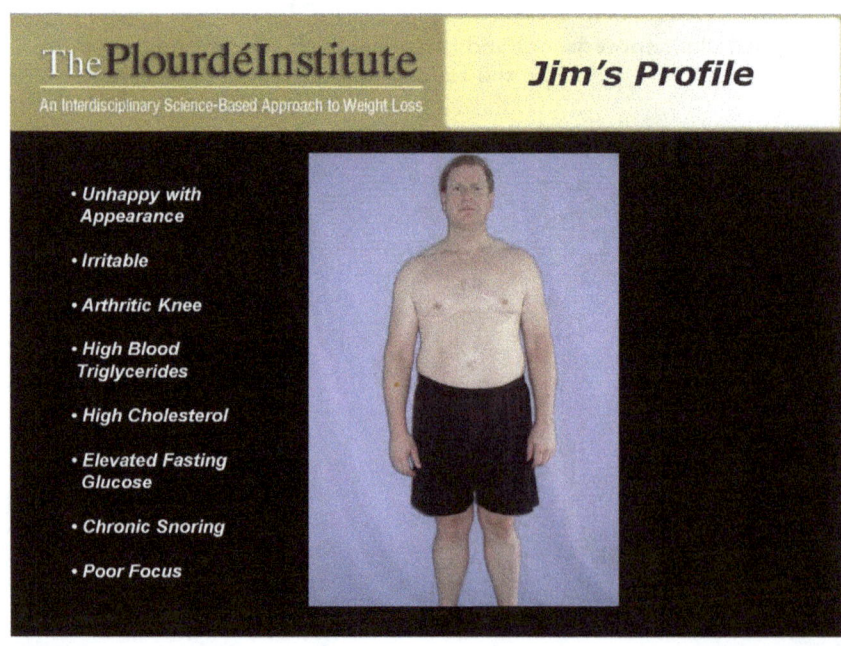

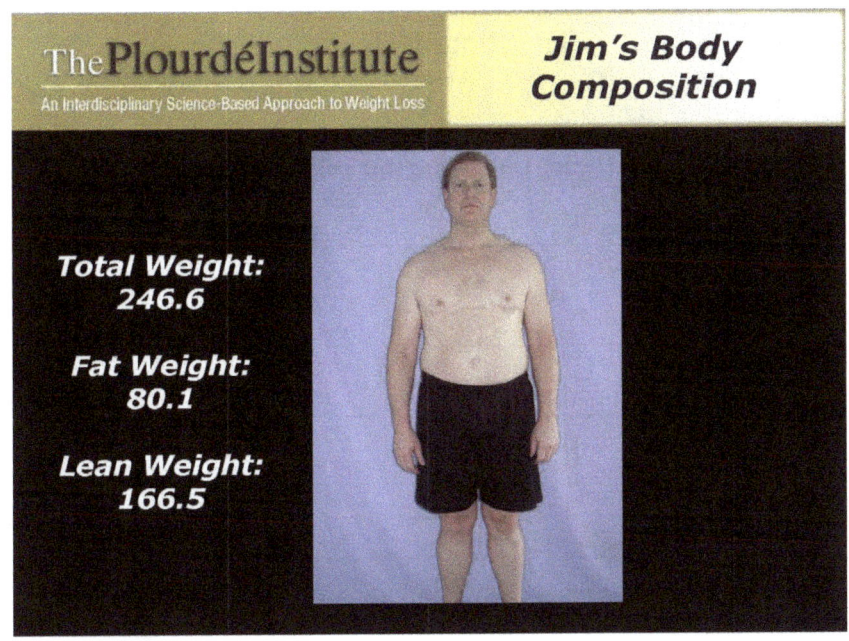

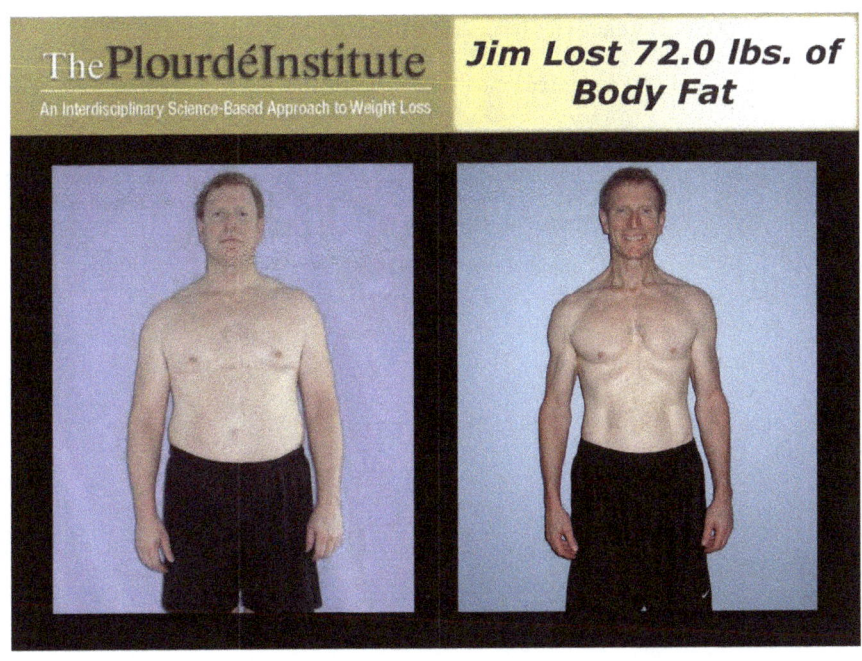

The Plourdé Institute
An Interdisciplinary Science-Based Approach to Weight Loss

Historical Evaluation of Adiposity

Name _____Jim_____   Date ___3/6/2009___

Condition of Adiposity	Baseline	Peak/ Current	Goal - 50%	Goal - 60%	Goal - 71%	Goal - 75%	Goal - 80%
Body Fat %	6.0	32.5	19.1	15.7	11.7	10.3	8.4
Fat Weight	11.1	80.1	40.1	32.0	23.2	20.0	16.0
Lean Weight	173.9	166.5	169.2	171.9	174.6	174.6	174.6
Total Weight	185.0	246.6	209.3	203.9	197.8	194.6	190.6
Age	17	55	55	55	55	55	55
# of Adipocytes	8.4	30.3	30.3	30.3	30.3	30.3	30.3

Fat Weight Increase of ___69.0___ lbs. = ___621.6___ %

Type of Lipogenesis =

(Type 1) Adipocyte Hypertrophy ☐

(Type 2) Adipocyte Hyperplastic Hypertrophy (Both Types) ☐

Fat Weight Reduction Goal: 40.1 lbs = 50.0 %
                              48.1 lbs = 60.0 %
                              56.9 lbs = 71.0 %
                              60.1 lbs = 75.0 %
                              64.1 lbs = 80.0 %

Estimated Range of Reduction Phase = __7-10__ months

Copyright © 2023 David Plourdé, Ph.D.

The Most Crucial Puzzle Piece: Your Meal Plan

BODY COMPOSITION PROGRESS CHART

CLIENT NAME: JIM **GOAL FAT WEIGHT: 6.1**

DATE	TOTAL WEIGHT	FAT WEIGHT	LEAN WEIGHT	FAT LOSS	% FAT LOSS	TOTAL FAT LOSS
3/6/2009	246.6	80.1	166.5			
4/3/2009	225.5	58.2	167.2	21.92	-27.3%	21.92
5/1/2009	210.9	43.1	167.8	15.12	-26.0%	37.04
5/29/2009	200.8	33.7	167.2	9.44	-21.9%	46.48
7/7/2009	191.9	23.1	168.7	10.53	-31.3%	57.02
8/14/2009	190.6	20.8	169.8	2.37	-10.2%	59.38
9/11/2009	186.6	16.7	169.9	4.02	-19.4%	63.40
10/9/2009	185.2	12.8	172.5	3.97	-23.7%	67.37
11/13/2009	182.9	10.4	172.5	2.39	-18.7%	69.77
2/12/2010	182.3	8.8	173.5	1.56	-15.0%	71.33
5/13/2010	182.2	8.6	173.6	0.23	-2.6%	71.56
8/13/2010	180.7	7.3	173.4	1.28	-14.9%	72.83
3/11/2011	182.9	9.1	173.9	-1.77	+24.2%	71.07
9/9/2011	179.9	8.1	171.9	1.03	-11.3%	72.09
3/9/2012	179.9	7.0	173.0	1.07	-13.3%	73.17
9/7/2012	179.3	7.1	172.2	-0.12	+1.8%	73.04
5/14/2013	186.4	12.8	173.6	-5.67	+79.8%	67.37
11/15/2013	182.2	9.0	173.2	3.73	-29.2%	71.10
5/15/2014	188.4	15.2	173.2	-6.18	+68.3%	64.92
11/14/2014	187.0	13.7	173.2	1.48	-9.7%	66.40
5/15/2015	183.6	9.7	173.9	4.02	-29.2%	70.42
11/13/2015	178.2	6.5	171.8	3.26	-33.5%	73.68
5/13/2016	179.0	7.2	171.8	-0.77	+12.0%	72.90
11/11/2016	180.1	9.0	171.0	-1.77	+24.4%	71.13
5/12/2017	179.2	8.2	171.0	0.79	-8.8%	71.92
11/17/2017	177.6	8.4	169.2	-0.15	+1.8%	71.78
2/16/2018	178.0	6.1	171.9	2.28	-27.2%	74.06
11/16/2018	177.4	6.2	171.2	-0.13	+2.1%	73.93
5/17/2019	177.3	6.1	171.2	0.15	-2.4%	74.08
11/15/2019	177.1	8.3	168.7	-2.28	+37.6%	71.80

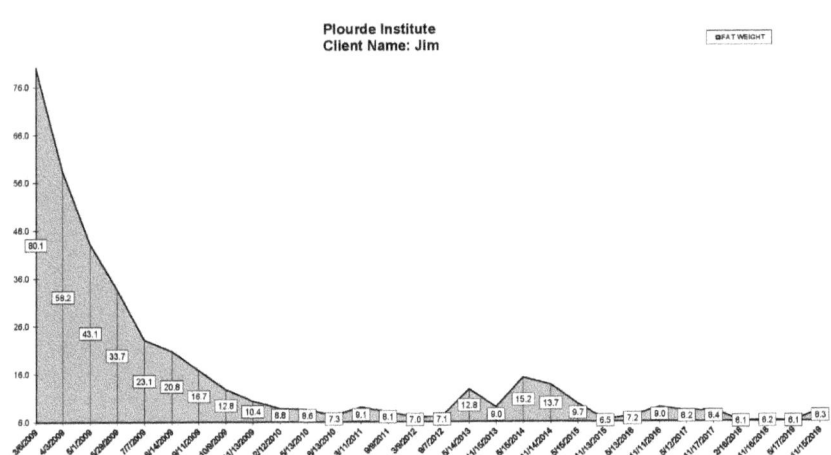

Plourde Institute
Client Name: Jim

When Jim was interviewed after his weight loss journey, he shared that the information that he learned at Plourdé is not available in our schools, from our physicians, or our churches. He said that the information AND the way it is organized will help you to put together all of the necessary pieces for a successful weight loss journey. It certainly produced a metamorphosis in his life he could not have imagined.

You can hear Jim's incredible story by scanning the QR code:

CHAPTER 8

I Hate to Break the Bad News . . .

I hate to break the bad news, but your nutrition supplements/vitamins are probably hampering your weight loss.

As I've made it clear thus far, my initial research objectives had to do with first developing a non-invasive technique to monitor Hormone-Sensitive Lipase and later, developing a full scientific method to control this enzyme. It was during this research that I learned just how sensitive HSL is: it's ridiculously sensitive! Let's take a closer look.

If you examine the Physicians' Desk Reference (PDR) database online, you will find that it contains a comprehensive list of medications approved by the United States Federal Drug Administration.

The pharmaceutical industry has made enormous strides in research and human health to help improve the lives of those who need medication. But here's a little-known FACT: practically every single medicine listed in the PDR has either a tablet base or capsule base of modified food starch—corn flour or powdered cellulose—potato flour. Many contain lactose or other "mystery" starches, such as

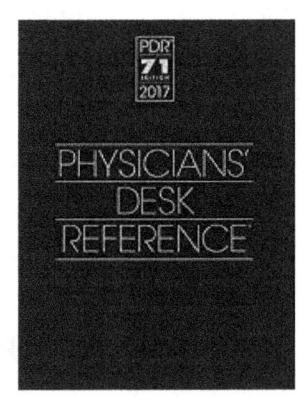

Source: Stock Photo

hypromellose, which is a semisynthetic starch replacement for gelatin. What I have seen firsthand while measuring cellular respiration in human subjects is that *even miniscule amounts of starch* in your nutrition supplements will evoke the secretion of insulin. The smallest secretions will trigger a suppression state of HSL in your fat cells.

Lipogenesis (Fat Synthesis)

Lipogenic State
During lipogenesis, HSL activity is suppressed and triglyceride degradation is inhibited. In the absence of fatty acid mobilization, new triglyceride formation continues and results in fat cell expansion and body weight increase.

Peak Fat Cell Weight: 1.4 micrograms

Plasma Membrane
FAT CELL EXPANSION
Nucleus
HSL
ENZYMATIC SUPPRESSION
NO DEGRADATION
Triglycerides
NEW TRIGLYCERIDE FORMATION

Credit: Created in BioRender. Plourde, D., Plourde, B. (2024) BioRender.com/b68u802

In application, if you take supplements containing these ingredients every day, you'll be triggering a suppression that lingers for days in **EACH INSTANCE**. So, if you've been super careful about watching your diet and making exercise a regular part of your routine, yet you have been dumbfounded by the lack of progress, you might need to pull up your chair and closely analyze your nutrition supplements.

I made clear observations in the third trial of my research, where we examined very carefully the presence of insidious sugars and starches and their impact on adipose tissue metabolism. This is the overall state of fat cells and whether they are creating new triglycerides and getting bigger or degrading triglycerides and getting smaller. The metabolic implications of having no knowledge of the presence of insidious carbohydrates in the first human trial versus having comprehensive knowledge and instruction to avoid these sneaky carbohydrates were notable.

A well-publicized weight loss program teaches a low-carb diet. The essence of the diet is very helpful. However, they make the claim that their supplement is an essential part to activating lipolysis in the human fat cell—a fancy term for influencing the fat cell to degrade or break the storage fat triglyceride, and subsequently directing the mobilization of fatty acids from the fat cell. If this were true, that would be wonderful. The problem is that the very basis of the capsule containing the minerals and other ingredients is *made of rice flour*. I'm in no way saying that their program is bad, I'm simply saying that their supplement contains an ingredient that will cause suppression of HSL. *People succeed in that program not because of the supplement, but rather in spite of it.*

You may be asking, "How could people on that weight loss program succeed if they were consuming a hidden starch every day?"

The answer is that when comparing the average American diet (high in sugar, starches, and fat) to a low carbohydrate diet, the cumulative metabolic benefit of the low carbohydrate diet is greater than the inhibiting effect of the rice flour-based capsule on HSL function. Without divulging intellectual property and trade secrets from my third trial, I can tell you with absolute certainty that the products you buy online, at the pharmacy, or at the store where you buy your vitamins are more often than not hindering your fat loss process every time you ingest them. Unfortunately, the nutrition supplement industry is chock-full of hyperbole. These manufacturers are guilty of making unsubstantiated claims and have done so for years. In no way am I suggesting that nutrition supplements are bad. As a matter of fact, I take them myself. However, the consumer is often the loser here, and unfortunately, it's not body fat they are losing!

The previous statement may seem hyperbolic, but it's not. In the third trial of my research, part of the information that I observed was correlated to changes in fat utilization and observable body fat weight loss plateaus. The data revealed that when subjects were given comprehensive guidance related to the avoidance of insidious sugars and starches (which included those found in nutrition supplements), body fat weight loss among those subjects was statistically greater, along with the rate of fatty acid utilization. This proved that insidious carbohydrates played an important role in when and where body fat weight loss plateaus occur.

What does this mean for you? It means that you should be looking for supplements that are free of insidious sugars and starches. **I suggest you look for nutrition supplements with a gelatin-based capsule.** Gelatin is comprised of proteins that come from collagen. Collagen is sourced from animals. However, almost entirely across the board, the nutrition supplement industry has replaced gelatin with starches such as rice flour, modified food starch, potato starch, and synthetic starches such as hypromellose for those people who prefer a vegetarian or vegan diet.

In my thousands upon thousands of lab tests, documenting with great detail the underlying chemical quality of what people are consuming from A-to-Z, I can tell you with authority that a gelatin-based supplement capsule is the superior way of delivering the intended ingredient because it does so *without the impending insulin secretion slowing your fat weight loss process down.*

You might also be asking the question, "Why do nutrition supplement companies use potato flour, corn flour, and other synthetic starches as the tableting and capsule base?"

My hypothesis is that it's because these substances are almost immediately chemically digested (broken down) and lead to a very fast rate of absorption. Here's the kicker, though: a fast rate of absorption is considered a good outcome, but the dirty little secret is that the underlying hidden starches absorb almost immediately *along with* the intended ingredients. These observations were confirmed through metabolic measurement tests that were conducted for all subjects in all three trials, taking into consideration the presence of these sneaky carbohydrates.

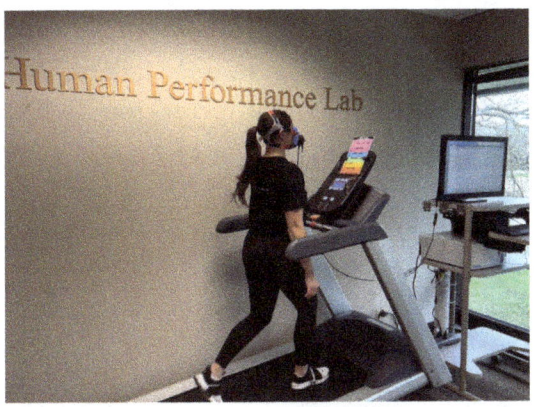

Source: The Plourdé Institute

I will provide instructions on how to access valuable resources at the end of the book in The Personal Invitation chapter. You'll learn how to get more clarifying information about nutrition, weight loss, and exercise on our website, but you will also have access to *supplements that are free of hidden sugars and starches* that will fill the micronutrient gaps that you need without triggering a suppression. Our supplement brand is called **Plourdé Nutrition**. I know this may sound like a shameless plug, and maybe it is, but I want to assure you that the supplements that we manufacture are controlled and free of these insidious carbohydrates that have been slowing you down for years. I'm hopeful that this new insight—along with other helpful tips—will alleviate confusion and ultimately free you from the frustration of unsuccessful weight loss.

▶▶▶ I'd like to help make this information come alive for you by sharing a client success story. I'd like to introduce you to Michael, a twenty-nine-year-old director of innovation for a tech company. Michael was winning in every way a person can win, except one: he was overweight. It wasn't because he wasn't trying to lose weight. He was striving to succeed in this area of his life through regular weight training, cardio exercise, eating a clean diet, and taking extensive amounts of nutrition supplements. In spite of all these efforts, this area of his life was an epic failure. We will get into that more later. Michael was referred to me by his family friend Paul, who was an out-of-state client of mine. Paul is a sixty-year-old business leader and he lost 52.3 pounds of fat, representing a 70.5 percent total body fat weight loss. Through the METHOD, he also gained 10 pounds of muscle.

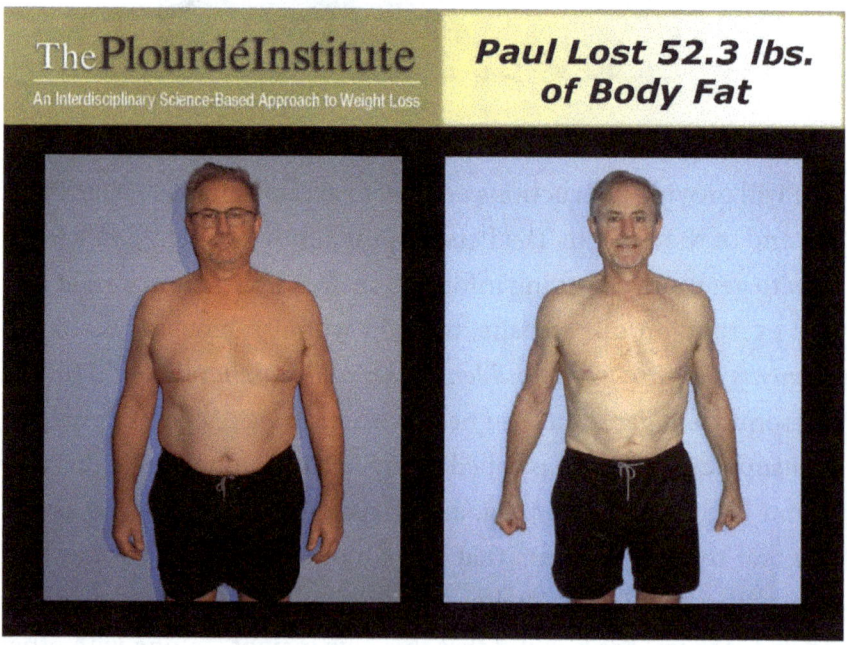

Inspired by this amazing outcome, Michael reached out to me and came in for an assessment on March 9, 2022. On that day, we learned that Michael's highest total weight was 240 pounds, with 79.1 pounds of body fat and 160.9 pounds of lean tissue. As previously mentioned, Michael was chasing his tail trying to achieve his body fat weight loss goals.

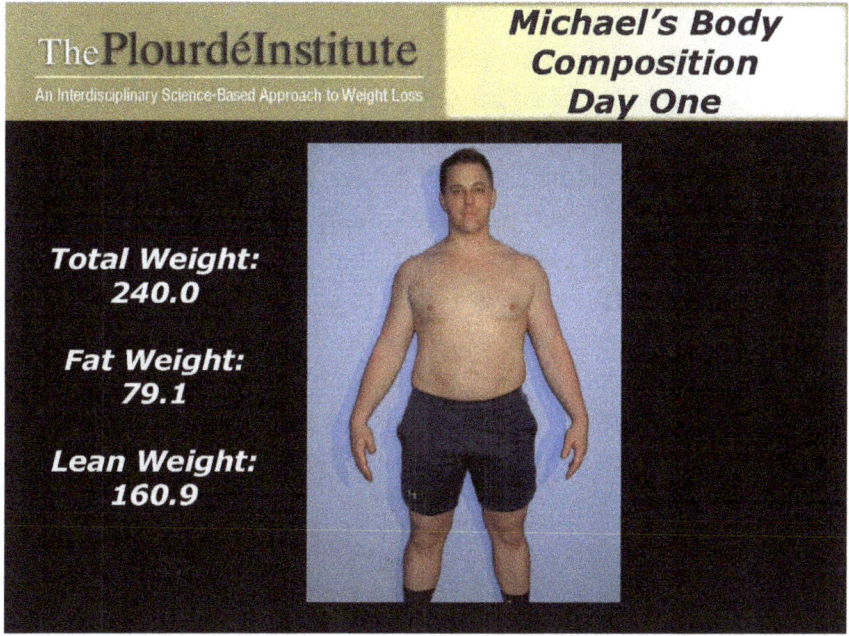

Michael complained of several "pains." First, he was frustrated with a lack of progress. On paper, he should have been losing body fat, but he wasn't. In fact, he was gaining body fat. An important note to make here is that Michael told me his primary source of nutrition information was "bro science videos" on YouTube made by so-called nutrition and fitness "experts" with zero science credentials.

His second "pain" was not knowing what to do or why to do it. Ultimately, his pain was confusion, and it was driving him crazy. He would incessantly watch those videos, taking copious notes, and follow suggested regimens to a T. Rather than losing fat, making progress, and feeling better, he felt more swollen, inflamed, and bloated, which led to a third "pain"—he was exhausted by what felt like a continual guessing game. In addition to these "primary pains," he also felt unhappy with his appearance, irritable, preoccupied with sugar cravings, and had poor focus.

So, in summary, Michael had a high clinical need for weight loss, had several psychological and emotional "pains" that created urgency, and an overall readiness for change. Right out of the gate, Michael learned that the HSL enzyme of his fat cells was in suppression, and until that enzyme mechanism was reactivated, there would be no real chance of substantial body fat weight loss. In preparation for his half-day assessment, I instructed him to bring all of the nutrition supplements that he was taking. Not just a list, but the actual bottles and containers so that I could thoroughly examine all of the ingredients lists. On the next couple of pages, you will find several supplement labels that have been recreated without the names or manufacturers, so as to not expose them directly, but rather shed light on the specific ingredients that trigger suppression.

To make this easier for you, the reader, I highlighted these ingredients in red.

Supplement Facts

Serving Size 7g
Servings per Container 30

	Amount per serving	%Daily Value
Calories	25	
Total Carbohydrate	4 g	1%**
Dietary Fiber	2 g	7%**
Total Sugars	0 g	†
Includes 0g Added Sugars		0%**
Protein	1 g	
Vitamin A	40 mcg	4%
Vitamin C	25 mg	28%
Vitamin K	45 mcg	38%
Calcium	30 mg	2%
Sodium	1 mg	6%
Iron	15 mg	1%
Potassium	120 mg	3%

Greens Blend — 4 g
Organic Wheat Grass, Organic Barley Grass, Organic Alfalfa Grass, Organic Spinach, Organic Spirulina, Organic Chlorella, Organic Broccoli †

Antioxidant Blend — 1.1 g †
Green Coffee Extract, *Green Tea Leaf Extract*, Broccoli Sprout, *Onion Extract*, *Apple Extract*, *Tomato*, Broccoli, *Camu Camu*, *Acerola Cherry Extract*, *Açai Berry*, *Turmeric*, *Garlic*, Basil, Oregano, *Cinnamon*, *Carrot*, *Elderberry*, *Mongosteen*, *Blackcurrant Extract*, *Blueberry Extract*, *Sweet Cherry*, *Raspberry*, Spinach, *Chokeberry*, Kale, *Blackberry*, *Bilberry Extract*, Brussel Sprouts, *Organic Rose Hips*, *Organic Pineapple*, *Organic Carrot*, *Acerola Cherry Extract*, *Organic Green Tea Leaf Extract*, *Organic Maca Root*, *Organic Açai Berry*, *Organic Beet Root*, *Organic Raspberry*

Fiber Blend — 467 mg †
Organic Flax Seed, *Organic Gum Acacia*

Digestive Enzyme & Pre/Probiotic Blend
F.O.S. (Fructooligosaccharide), Amylase (*Aspergillus oryzae*), Protease (*Aspergillus oryzae*), Lipase (*Aspergillus niger*), Lactase (*Aspergillus oryzae*), Cellulase (*Trichoderma reesei*), Lactobacillus acidophilus †

**Percent Daily Values are based on a 2,000 calorie diet.   †Daily Value not established

Other Ingredients: *Natural Flavor*, Citric Acid, *Fruit and Vegetable Juice for Color*, Organic Peppermint Leaf, *Stevia Leaf Extract*, *Silica*.

Source: The Plourdé Institute
(label re-created for the purpose of this book)

Supplement Facts

Servings Per Container: 30
Serving Size: 1 Scoop (5.5 g)

Amount Per Serving	% Daily Value
Calories 15	
Total Carbohydrate 2 g	<1%**
Dietary Fiber <1 g	3%**
Vitamin C (as magnesium ascorbate) 60 mg	100%
Magnesium (as magnesium ascorbate) 20 mg	5%
Beets Blend 4.3 g	†
Non-GMO Beet root juice powder (Beta vulgaris L.), *Non-GMO Organic fermented Beet root juice powder (Beta vulgaris L.)*,	

**Percent Daily Values are based on a 2,000 Calorie diet.
†Daily Value not established.

Other Ingredients: *Guar gum*, citric acid, *natural flavor*, *silica* & *rebaudioside-A*.

Source: The Plourdé Institute
(label re-created for the purpose of this book)

Nutrition Facts

53 servings per container
Serving size   33 g (About 1 Scoop)

Amount per serving
Calories   **120**

	% Daily Value*
Total Fat 0.5g	1%
Cholesterol 15mg	5%
Sodium 230mg	10%
Total Carbohydrate 3g	1%
Dietary Fiber 1g	4%
Total Sugars 1g	
Includes 0g Added Sugars	0%
Protein 24g	48%
Calcium 500mg	40%
Magnesium 85mg	20%
Zinc 11mg	100%

Not a significant source of saturated fat, trans fat, vitamin D, iron and potassium.

*The % Daily Value tells you how much a nutrient in a serving of food contributes to a daily diet. 2,000 calories a day is used for general nutrition advice.

INGREDIENTS: *Micellar Casein*, *Natural and Artificial Flavor*, Inulin, Salt, *Gum Blend (Guar Gum, Gum Acacia, Xanthan Gum)*, Sunflower and/or Soy Lecithin, Magnesium Oxide, Sucralose, Zinc Sulfate Monohydrate.

CONTAINS: MILK AND SOY.

Source: The Plourdé Institute
(label re-created for the purpose of this book)

Nutrition Facts

40 servings per container
Serving size   40 g (About 1 Scoop)

Amount per serving
Calories **140**

% Daily Value*

Total Fat 1g	1%
Saturated Fat 0.5g	3%
Cholesterol 35mg	12%
Sodium 160mg	7%
Total Carbohydrate 3g	1%
Total Sugars 1g	
Protein 30g	60%
Calcium 150mg	10%
Potassium 180mg	4%

Not a significant source of trans fat, dietary fiber, added sugars, vitamin D and iron.

*The % Daily Value tells you how much a nutrient in a serving of food contributes to a daily diet. 2,000 calories a day is used for general nutrition advice.

INGREDIENTS: Hydrolyzed Whey Protein Isolate, Branched Chain Amino Acids (L-Leucine, L-Isoleucine, L-Valine), *Natural and Artificial Flavor*, Sunflower and/or Soy Lecithin, Creamer (Sunflower Oil, *Maltodextrin*, *Modified Food Starch*, Dipotassium Phosphate, Tricalcium Phosphate, Tocopherols), Salt, *Guar Gum*, Sucralose, Acesulfame Potassium.

CONTAINS: MILK AND SOY.

Source: The Plourdé Institute
(label re-created for the purpose of this book)

I'm in no way suggesting these supplements are bad or unhealthy. The truth is, they're good, but as you will soon find out, if a person's goal is to achieve substantial fat weight loss, but they are consistently consuming these insidious forms of sugar and starch, the subsequent insulin secretion will render the fat cells incapable of mobilizing fatty acids for days each time they're ingested. Moreover, in this state of suppression, fat cells synthesize new triglyceride, causing fat cell weight and body fat weight to go up. And that's precisely what Michael was experiencing and why, although he was following a relatively clean diet and exercising regularly, his body was resisting fat loss.

After onboarding Michael, I also instructed him to stop taking those previously mentioned supplements. I think it's important to note here that had he followed my instructions on the meal plan and exercise prescriptions, but had continued to take the supplements, the program would not have worked. He realized that as I pointed it out to him in a laboratory setting. Adipose tissue metabolism had completely changed from fatty acids being unavailable for cellular respiration and the body defaulting to glucose utilization to the converse. Fat became the primary source of fuel in cellular respiration. This wasn't a theoretical concept; Michael personally witnessed this, and with body composition testing conducted in the BOD POD every four weeks, he experienced mathematically linear body fat weight loss. You can see his body composition spreadsheet ahead:

The Plourdé Institute
An Interdisciplinary Science-Based Approach to Weight Loss

BODY COMPOSITION PROGRESS CHART							
CLIENT NAME: MICHAEL				GOAL FAT WEIGHT: 15.8			
DATE	TOTAL WEIGHT	FAT WEIGHT	LEAN WEIGHT	FAT LOSS	% FAT LOSS		TOTAL FAT LOSS
1/1/2022	240.0	79.1	160.9				
3/9/2022	235.0	74.1	160.9	5.07	-6.4%		5.07
4/8/2022	212.4	50.3	162.1	23.77	-32.1%		28.84
5/6/2022	202.8	37.8	165.0	12.45	-24.8%		41.29
6/9/2022	193.0	26.9	166.1	10.90	-28.8%		52.19
7/15/2022	185.9	17.8	168.1	9.17	-34.0%		61.35
9/7/2022	187.9	15.3	172.6	2.52	-14.2%		63.88

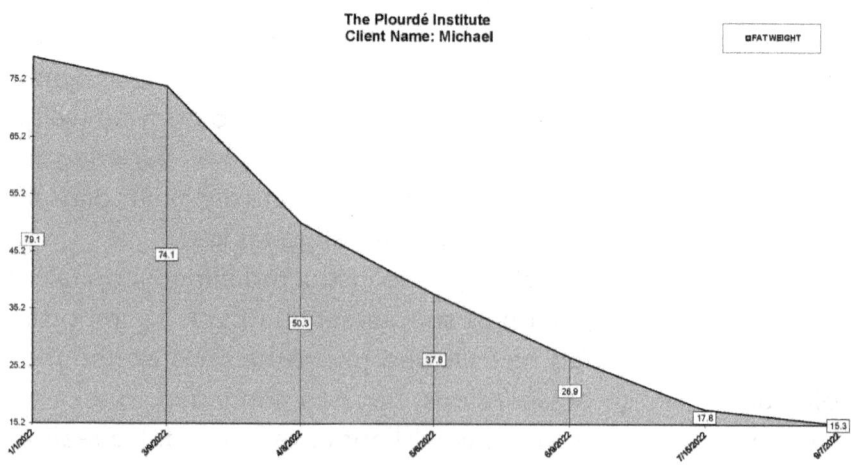

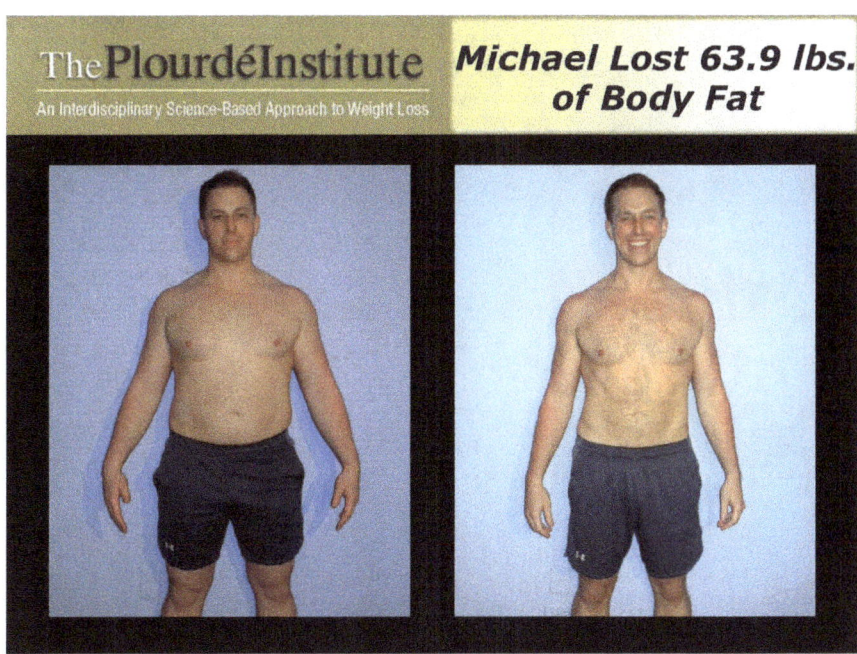

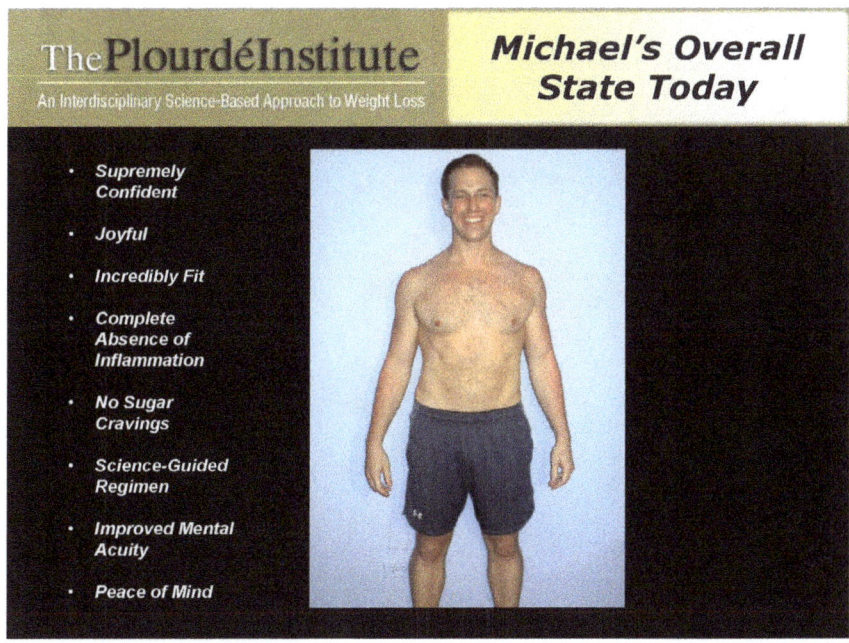

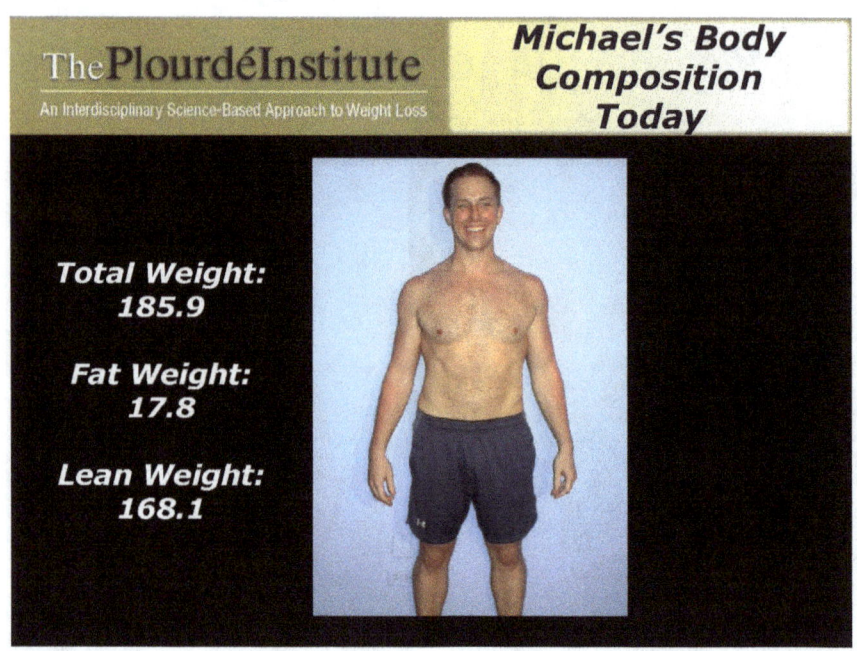

The Plourdé Institute
An Interdisciplinary Science-Based Approach to Weight Loss

Historical Evaluation of Adiposity

Name _____Michael_____   Date ___3/9/2022___

Condition of Adiposity	Baseline	Peak	Current	Goal - 50%	Goal - 60%	Goal - 71%	Goal - 75%	Goal - 80%
Body Fat %	10.0	32.9	31.5	19.5	16.0	12.0	10.5	8.6
Fat Weight	18.5	79.1	74.2	39.6	31.6	22.9	19.8	15.8
Lean Weight	166.5	160.9	160.9	163.6	166.3	169.0	169.0	169.0
Total Weight	185.0	240.0	235.1	203.2	197.9	191.9	188.8	184.8
Age	19	29	30	30	30	30	30	30
# of Adipocytes	14.0	29.9	29.9	29.9	29.9	29.9	29.9	29.9

Fat Weight Increase of ___60.6___ lbs. = ___327.6___ %

Type of Lipogenesis =

(Type 1) Adipocyte Hypertrophy ☐

(Type 2) Adipocyte Hyperplastic Hypertrophy (Both Types) ☐

Fat Weight Reduction Goal: 34.7 lbs = 46.7 %
                              42.6 lbs = 57.4 %
                              51.3 lbs = 69.1 %
                              54.4 lbs = 73.3 %
                              58.4 lbs = 78.7 %

Estimated Range of Reduction Phase = __9-11__ months

Copyright © 2023 David Plourdé, Ph.D.

www.theplourdeinstitute.com
901 Warrenville Road, Suite 110, Lisle, Illinois, 60532   630.769.0776

In conclusion, although the name of this chapter is, "I Hate to Break the Bad News . . .," there is inherently good news for you here. On March 9, 2022, Michael's tail chase ended. We replaced his confusion, frustration, and exhaustion with peace of mind and clarity. Just like him, your tail chase ends now! If you carefully follow my instructions, you will find the freedom, better health, joy, and self-respect that you are seeking. I feel so honored and privileged to take you by the hand (albeit through my book) and deliver this incredible outcome for you. ▶▶▶

Watch Michael's Incredible Story Here:

CHAPTER 9

Everything You Think You Know About Exercise Is Wrong!

I know that the title of this chapter may seem hyperbolic. If I hadn't seen thousands of people exercise themselves to higher levels of body fat, maybe I wouldn't believe it either. In this chapter, I will systematically teach you the science of how to exercise for optimum fat loss. This is an essential piece to solving your weight loss puzzle. Let's do this!

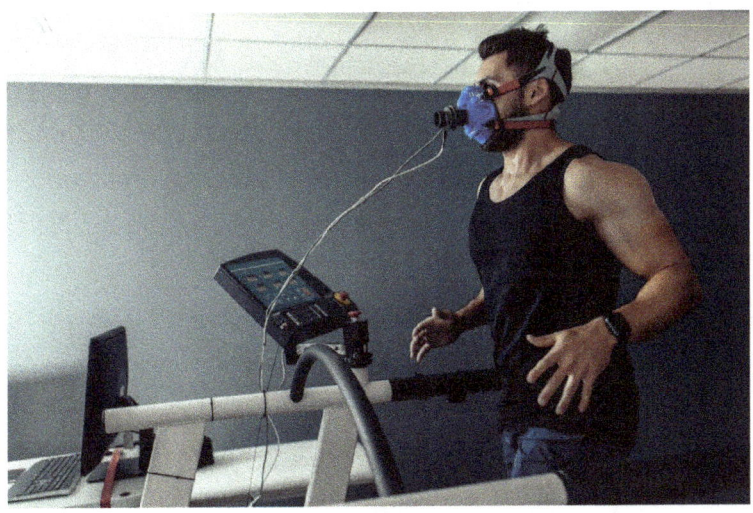

Source: Texas A&M University — Central Texas Website
(Exercise Physiology & Human Performance, 2024)

One of the biggest secrets to successful weight loss is found in the underlying fact that there are three distinctly different types of muscle fiber that control fuel utilization. Think of it as first, second, and third gear muscle fibers. Also known as red slow twitch, red fast twitch, and white fast twitch muscle fibers, respectively.

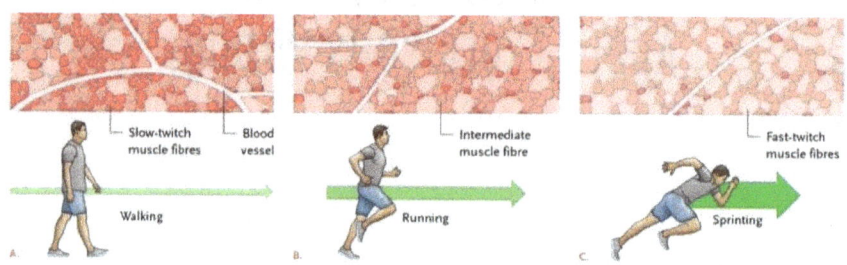

Source: *Human Biology, Anatomy & Physiology for the Health Sciences, 2nd Edition*
Author: Wendi A. Roscoe
Publisher: Top Hat
(Roscoe, 2019)

First gear muscle fibers *utilize fatty acids exclusively. They are red in color and contain a red oxygen-binding pigment called myoglobin. Myoglobin is similar to hemoglobin, an oxygen-binding protein in the bloodstream that helps to transport oxygen. This is an important detail, because without myoglobin in the muscle fiber, oxygen cannot enter the muscle cell, and unless oxygen is present, fatty acids CANNOT be utilized as a fuel source.*

Second gear muscle fibers, also called red fast twitch muscle fibers, are different from first gear muscle fibers in that they can adapt from the utilization of fatty acids to the utilization of glucose. *So, second gear muscle fibers can use fat* **or** *sugar for fuel in cellular respiration. Like first gear muscle fibers, they are red in color and contain the red oxygen-binding pigment called myoglobin.*

Third gear muscle fibers are called white fast twitch fibers. They are uniquely different in that they preclude the utilization of fatty acids and *drive cellular work exclusively on glucose (sugar) in the absence of oxygen.* That's because white fast twitch fibers do not contain the red oxygen binding protein myoglobin.

Let me bring this to life for you by sharing something I learned from my clinical experience. In the course of thousands of VO2 max stress tests, monitoring untrained to moderately trained overweight human subjects who ate the standard American diet, I've made the following observations:

At 2.0 to 2.4 miles per hour (mph) on a treadmill, the muscle fibers use primarily fat. However, when the body shifts to a slow jog at 4.0 to 4.5 mph, the muscle fibers begin pivoting to the utilization of glucose. By the time a person is moving at 5 or 6 mph or faster, the muscles will have switched entirely to the utilization of glucose. Practically speaking, what does this mean for you? **Most, if not all, of the exercise you've ever done for weight loss, you've done wrong—metabolically speaking.**

YOUR NEW METABOLICALLY-CONTROLLED EXERCISE PRESCRIPTION:
Ideally, walking on a treadmill.

Here is a chart outlining my recommendations for the speed at which you should be walking:

Height	Walking Speed (miles per hour)
Up to 5'0" ($\leq$ 60 inches)	1.8 to 2.2
5'1" to 5'8" (61-68 inches)	2.2 to 2.4
5'9" to 6'0" (69-72 inches)	2.4
6'1" to 6'5" (73-77 inches)	2.6 to 3.0
6'6" and taller (78+ inches)	3.0 to 3.2

The essence here is that the muscles are moving at a slow rate of speed. This will activate first and second gear muscle fibers to utilize exclusively fatty acids.

If you walk markedly more vigorously than these speeds, you might as well hang up your gym shoes and go home, because third gear muscle fibers, also known as white fast twitch muscle fibers, lack the oxygen binding myoglobin. Therefore, oxygen cannot enter the muscle cell. Without oxygen present, fatty acids cannot be utilized in cellular respiration, and the body defaults to the utilization of glucose.

The problem with this is that inevitably, a person will exhaust the glycogen storage (the polymers or chains of glucose) in the muscle fibers. The feeding centers of the brain will recognize this fuel depletion and direct a hunger for sugar and starches in a manner you can't predict, control, or satisfy. This hunger response is purely physiological in nature. It is NOT a discipline problem. Ironically, you will exercise yourself into a higher level of body fat.

As you contemplate your previous weight loss efforts, as well as your exercise regimen, I'm sure you can recall a time when you had a sudden taste for Mexican food, French fries, candy, or chips following a rigorous exercise session. I'm hoping that you're connecting the dots. Among the people that I have guided through our weight loss program, essentially all of them have confessed these types of stories and have breathed a huge sigh of relief when I explained the details of their exercise prescription.

See the diagram of the hypothalamus along with the feeding centers and satiety center below:

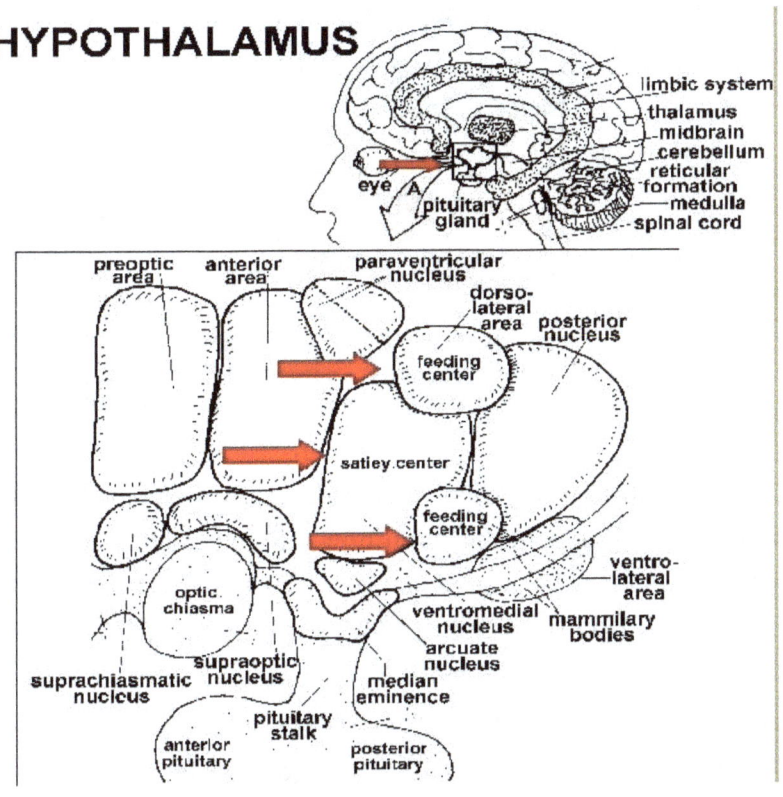

Source: (Kapit, Macey, and Meisami, 1987)

Now, we move onto the next aspect of your treadmill exercise prescription: incline level. Walking at a speed of 2.4 mph, raise the incline to a level that coincides with the rate of perceived exertion of 12 on the Borg scale.

See the diagram of the **Borg scale** below:

BORG SCALE PERCEIVED EXERTION	
6	
7	VERY, VERY LIGHT
8	
9	VERY LIGHT
10	
11	FAIRLY LIGHT
12	
13	SOMEWHAT HARD
14	
15	HARD
16	
17	VERY HARD
18	
19	VERY, VERY HARD

Source: The Plourdé Institute based upon
The Borg RPE Scale: "Borg, G. (1998).
Borg's perceived exertion and pain scales. Human Kinetics")

You will notice that when you're walking at speeds ranging from 1.8 to 2.6 mph, depending upon how tall you are, the incline will make the exercise far more vigorous. **Here's the important point**: *when you raise the incline on the treadmill, the muscles still continue to move at the same speed, but the calorie expenditure increases exponentially. This increase in calorie expenditure will come exclusively from the utilization of fatty acids and not glucose, because the muscles are* **still moving at the same speed** *that exclusively activates the red slow twitch and red fast twitch muscle fibers.*

Think about it. When the HSL enzyme is re-activated in the fat cell, you unlock the fat cells for continuous mobilization of fatty acids. When the fatty acids exit the fat cell, they hit the bloodstream and circulate. Under these conditions of metabolically-controlled exercise, the **muscle fibers will take up the fatty acids from the bloodstream and utilize them at four to six times the normal rate with little to no utilization of glucose.** The astounding fact is that you will have **no sugar cravings** when exercising this way. Also, body fat weight loss will occur at a mathematically linear rate on a monthly basis when guided by the scientific principles outlined in this book. This will translate to 10 to 14 percent body fat weight loss per month every single month until a biological plateau in body fat weight loss occurs.

Next, the duration of exercise should range anywhere from thirty to sixty continuous minutes. The exception of course would be if you're tired or sore. In these circumstances, drop the incline to a level that is comfortable and maintain a 12 at all times on the Borg scale for perceived exertion. **Less is more.** The exercise should not be hard. In fact, exercising too vigorously has probably played a major role in your lack of successful body fat weight loss your entire adult life.

What about **heart rate**? First of all, the exercise prescription is *not heart rate driven*, **it is metabolism driven**. Meaning, that exercise exertion is pinpointed to the maximum efficiency of fatty acid utilization (and the exclusion of glucose utilization), not a specific heart rate. Certain blood pressure medications, called beta blockers, prevent the heart rate from climbing in a normal fashion for the purposes of decreasing myocardial oxygen demand in patients with coronary artery disease or hypertension. For some implementing these instructions, your heart rate will climb higher than what you may have been used to. This is a very individualized aspect of the exercise prescription that can only be specified from an individual laboratory experience. If you were a private client and I was conducting a VO2 max stress test for you, the specific heart rate range would be included here, but we don't have that luxury. I think it's important to note that your overall perceived exertion on the Borg scale is far more important than a specific heart rate. Your maximum heart rate can be estimated by the following equation:

These calculations will give you a general sense of where your heart rate range may fall.

220 minus your age = X	X multiplied by .6 = heart rate that is 60% of predicted max heart rate
220 minus your age = X	X multiplied by .7 = heart rate that is 70% of predicted max heart rate
220 minus your age = X	X multiplied by .75 = heart rate that is 75% of predicted max heart rate

Remember, the most important factor is to maintain a perceived exertion of 12 for both breathing and overall body exertion.

It is best for you to **fulfill the exercise prescription first thing in the morning**, preferably in a fasting state. If you exercise in the late afternoon or evening, the epinephrine, norepinephrine, and growth hormone responses will cause brain arousal that may prevent you from getting to sleep or preventing deep sleep, causing you to feel sleep deprivation the following day. This will result in elevated cortisol, a stress hormone that will trigger a suppression in your fat cells similar to that of insulin, thus defaulting to the utilization of glucose.

If it is not possible to exercise in the morning, early afternoon is acceptable. For some of you, this won't be possible either. Do the best you can with the timing of exercise.

A note about overuse injuries, joint replacements, cardiovascular disease, pulmonary disorders, and certain medications: if any of these apply to you, you will need to see an exercise physiologist and medical doctor to confirm the appropriate level and type of exercise for you.

A Word to Those Who Are Disabled

If you have a disability that renders you incapable of walking or using your lower limbs, you can still be successful in weight loss.

▶▶▶ Let me share a very personal story: Pastor John arrived at The Plourdé Institute in September 2012. We conducted an assessment, evaluating the pastor's clinical need for weight loss as well as his psychological and emotional readiness for change. He was a great candidate; however, he was in a wheelchair and could not exercise in conventional ways.

I prescribed pool exercise for the pastor exclusively. Although he was unable to walk, he was able to lose over one hundred pounds of body fat. It was truly a blessing and a miracle for both of us to see this happen. I'm including his story for those of you who may have a similar circumstance.

The general exercise recommendations for the pastor involved any movements he could conduct with the resistance of water at a perceived exertion of 12 on the Borg scale. Initially, his exercise duration was fifteen minutes, but over the course of his program, the duration extended to one hour. ▶▶▶

Let me remind you that **your diet is 80 percent of the equation**, and if you are mindful of being under your calorie targets slightly, your body *will allow for body fat weight loss, even in the absence of conventional exercise.* Many exercises can be conducted in a wheelchair using your arms, shoulders, chest, and back muscles. If this is your situation, I recommend that you seek out a knowledgeable, highly trained personal trainer who is experienced in working with people who are in a wheelchair. Keep in mind that your exercise should never exceed a 12 on the Borg scale because the muscle fibers will switch to glucose utilization, sending you into a cycle of hunger that will undermine everything we are trying to accomplish.

A Word about High Intensity Exercise

High intensity exercise tends to activate white fast twitch muscle fibers, and as I have mentioned previously, we know that these muscle fibers utilize sugar. Having said that, it's my custom not to add weight training to a client's overall program until they have lost the majority of their body fat and entered into a plateau. Here's why: I'll demonstrate this aspect of my METHOD by sharing a story.

▶▶▶ Shannon, from the western suburbs of Chicago, was in her mid- to late-fifties and was losing more than 10 percent of her body fat on a monthly basis. Everything about her program was happening quite smoothly. Her metabolism measurements showed high rates of fat utilization, BOD POD tests showed significant fat loss, and she was thrilled with the results.

That all suddenly and mysteriously changed. Her body fat weight loss seemed to stall and her fat utilization dropped significantly. Baffled by this observation, I asked her a question, "Are you doing any exercise in addition to what I have prescribed?"

She answered, "As a matter of fact, yes."

So, I asked her what she was doing. She went on to share that she was playing Paddle, an outdoor ice tennis game, three to five nights per week. It's an activity that involves quick starts and stops. In other words, it's an anaerobic activity that activates white fast twitch muscle fibers that utilize glucose exclusively. ▶▶▶

I want to say that there is nothing inherently wrong with this. However, when a person follows THE PLOURDE METHOD℠ and fat cells are free of suppression and continuously mobilizing fatty acids, but the muscle fibers have switched to utilizing exclusively sugar, the fatty acids cannot enter the muscle fiber and continue to circulate in the bloodstream. At this point, they become available for a process called reesterification. This means fat is mobilized from one fat cell, hits the bloodstream, and circulates, but does not get utilized and therefore reforms as a triglyceride (storage fat) in a different fat cell somewhere else in the body. In application, it's the reason why I don't add weight training until body fat weight loss has plateaued. If the body sculpting layer of enhancement is added too soon, it definitely slows down the weight loss process. Unless a person is a scientist operating in a laboratory setting, there is no way to know this. This may be one explanation why your previous weight loss efforts have been so frustrating.

Here's a quick summary to make sure you maximize fat utilization and spare muscle glycogen:

1. **Follow the meal plan as prescribed and remember to entirely eliminate both obvious and insidious sugars and starches.** When you ingest either an obvious or an insidious source of sugar or starch, the fat cells are locked down for days, only allowing for the synthesis of new fat. This means that body fat weight actually goes up after eating sugar or starch. You do not merely just stop losing weight, it actually reverses the process, and you start gaining!

2. **Eat on a schedule of two and a half hour intervals.** This will prevent the body from going into gluconeogenesis or the utilization of proteins from muscles, organs, and other lean tissues.

3. **Walk on the treadmill exclusively, as prescribed above**, until your body fat weight loss plateaus as it relates to your personal predicted body fat loss calculation.

4. **Metabolically-controlled weight training should not be incorporated until after your body fat weight loss has plateaued.**

Let me illustrate the power of metabolically-controlled exercise with client case studies Scott and Chuck:

▶▶▶ Scott was forty-nine years old when we first met. He is a majority shareholder and president of an automotive car dealership business. This is a very well-known car dealership in the Chicago area that's been around for over forty years. Scott was referred to me by one of his best friends, Rick, who is a successful attorney and professor of law at one of the nation›s leading law schools.

Scott arrived at The Plourdé Institute on October 20, 2010, for a weight loss assessment. His highest body weight occurred three years prior, at which point his total weight was 260 pounds with 107.3 pounds of body fat weight and 152.7 pounds of lean tissue. On the day of the assessment, his total weight was 246.9, with 94.2 pounds of fat and 152.7 pounds of muscle. The thought of turning fifty years old in his current state was nothing short of disgusting to him!

Scott suffered from chronic snoring and obstructive sleep apnea. He also had difficulty breathing because he had an obstructed diaphragm from massive intra-abdominal body fat. He struggled with stiffness, swelling, fatigue, and a lack of mental clarity. The cumulative mass of his overall pain was the necessary prerequisite that spurred his psychological and emotional readiness for change. He was entirely ready to embrace THE PLOURDE METHOD[SM].

On that day, we marked out a regimen, including prescribed diet, metabolically-controlled exercise, specific accountability structures, as well as a forecast of body fat weight loss of 14 percent per month. See Scott's body composition spreadsheet in the pages ahead outlining a body fat weight loss of 20 percent per month for the first five months. I think it's important that I point out that I have a philosophy in my practice: never exaggerate; seek always to under promise and overdeliver. Exaggerating never helps anyone, especially when the subject is as sensitive as this one. Scott's body fat weight went from 94.2 pounds to 13.9 pounds in the course of nine months.

The part of Scott's story that is of particular importance to this chapter was that before meeting me he was a weekend warrior avid bicyclist. It would not be uncommon for Scott to bike one hundred miles in a single ride on the weekend and as many as three hundred miles on special occasions. Despite his rigorous discipline for regular exercise, he was entirely incapable of having any substantial body fat loss. He was baffled by the lack of progress. During his assessment, Scott underwent a VO2 max stress test and learned that all of the exercise he had ever performed had been conducted entirely metabolically wrong. His muscle fibers utilized exclusively glucose in the muscle contractions without fatty acid utilization. This explains why, after exercising, he would have a hunger for sugars and starches that he could not predict, control, or satisfy.

After being presented with THE PLOURDE METHOD[SM] in a concise and straightforward manner, he decided to move forward with the program and experienced a profound paradigm shift: he had absolutely no cravings for sugars or starches, and his body fat weight loss occurred in an almost effortless fashion. You can hear Scott's personal experience where he differentiates between performance training and exercising for body fat weight loss. I think you'll find his story particularly eye-opening and I hope you take time to watch: ▶▶▶

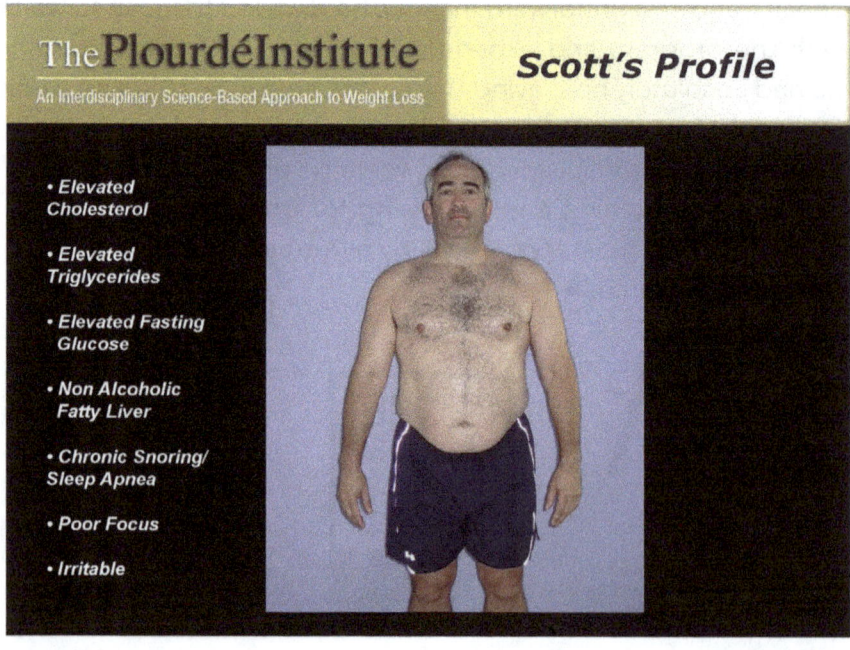

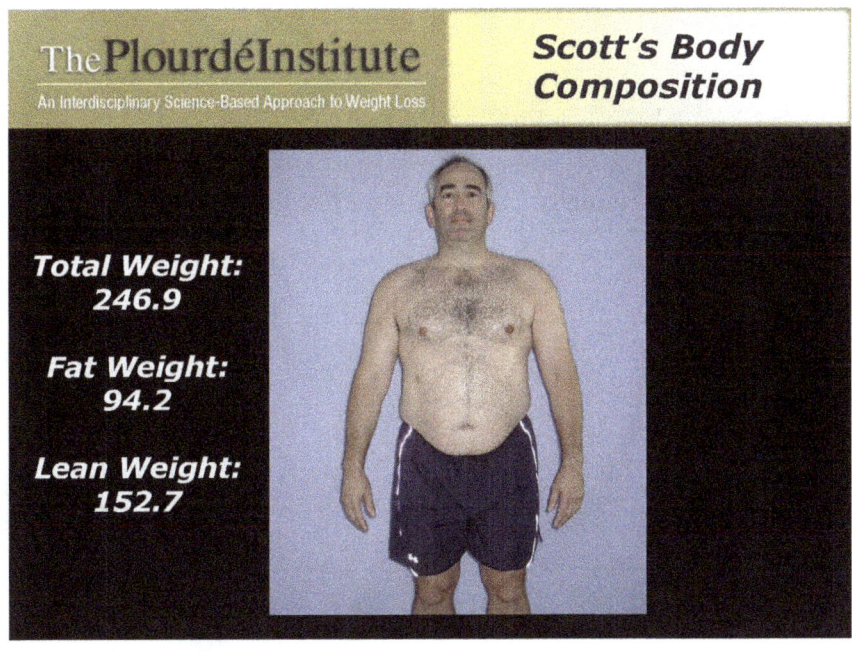

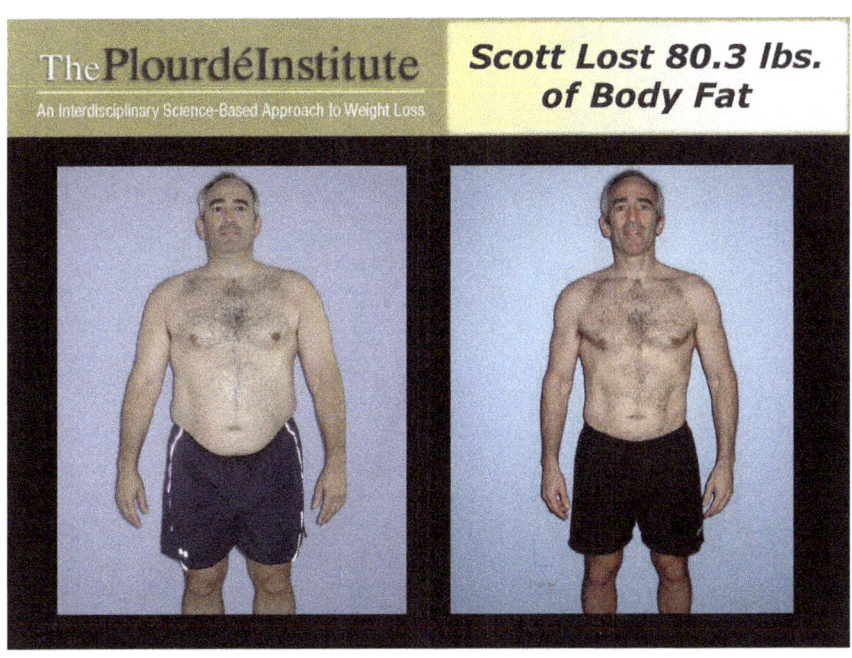

The Plourdé Institute
An Interdisciplinary Science-Based Approach to Weight Loss

Historical Evaluation of Adiposity

Name ____Scott____   Date ___3/23/2011___

Condition of Adiposity	Baseline	Peak	Current	Goal - 50%	Goal - 60%	Goal - 71%	Goal - 75%	Goal - 80%
Body Fat %	18.0	41.1	38.0	25.5	21.2	16.1	14.2	11.7
Fat Weight	32.0	106.9	93.8	53.5	42.8	31.0	26.7	21.4
Lean Weight	155.0	153.1	153.1	155.8	158.5	161.2	161.2	161.2
Total Weight	190.0	260.0	246.9	209.3	201.3	192.2	187.9	182.6
Age	17	46	49	49	49	49	49	49
# of Adipocytes	24.2	40.4	40.4	40.4	40.4	40.4	40.4	40.4

Fat Weight Increase of ___74.9___ lbs. = ___234.1___ %

Type of Lipogenesis =

(Type 1) Adipocyte Hypertrophy ☐

(Type 2) Adipocyte Hyperplastic Hypertrophy (Both Types) ☐

Fat Weight Reduction Goal: 40.4 lbs   =   43.0 %
                              51.0 lbs   =   54.4 %
                              62.8 lbs   =   66.9 %
                              67.7 lbs   =   71.5 %
                              72.4 lbs   =   77.2 %

Estimated Range of Reduction Phase = __7-10__ months

Copyright © 2023 David Plourdé, Ph.D.

The Plourdé Institute
An Interdisciplinary Science-Based Approach to Weight Loss

BODY COMPOSITION PROGRESS CHART

CLIENT NAME: SCOTT **GOAL FAT WEIGHT: 13.9**

DATE	TOTAL WEIGHT	FAT WEIGHT	LEAN WEIGHT	FAT LOSS	% FAT LOSS	TOTAL FAT LOSS
10/20/2007	260.0	107.3	152.7			
10/20/2010	246.9	94.2	152.7	13.06	-12.2%	13.06
11/23/2010	222.0	68.0	154.0	26.23	-27.8%	39.30
12/14/2010	213.6	57.6	156.0	10.38	-15.3%	49.68
1/12/2011	202.8	44.6	158.2	12.96	-22.5%	62.64
2/15/2011	194.8	33.9	160.9	10.71	-24.0%	73.36
3/15/2011	189.4	27.2	162.2	6.75	-19.9%	80.11
4/12/2011	186.9	24.0	162.9	3.20	-11.8%	83.31
5/12/2011	183.9	18.5	165.4	5.53	-23.0%	88.83
6/15/2011	183.0	17.4	165.6	1.03	-5.6%	89.86
8/30/2011	180.6	13.9	166.7	3.53	-20.2%	93.39
12/8/2011	180.2	15.8	164.4	-1.88	+13.5%	91.51
6/20/2012	180.1	15.1	165.0	0.69	-4.4%	92.21

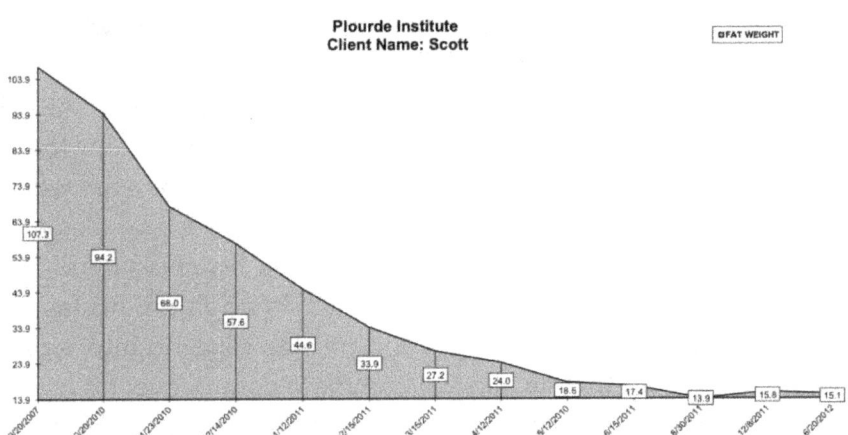

Let's take a look at another client success story where metabolically-controlled exercise played a major role:

▶▶▶ Chuck is sixty years old. He runs a mortgage company and is also a commercial real estate owner. He's married to his lovely wife, Lisa, and has two amazing kids who are flourishing. He played football in high school and college as a defensive back and had always been proud of his physique. Chuck has succeeded in every way a person can succeed.

Throughout his life, as he aged, he had always prioritized exercise, perhaps to a fault. Chuck maintained several gym memberships, ran multiple times a week, lifted heavy weights, experimented with high-intensity interval training (HIIT), and was a self-proclaimed 'gym rat.' His body was breaking down and he was suffering from multiple overuse injuries. At one point, Chuck suffered a ruptured bicep and had to undergo surgery where he could not exercise for three to four months.

At that moment, he was disgusted with his appearance. At 218 pounds, this was his all-time highest weight, and he later found out that his body fat level was 69.8 pounds. Perhaps even worse than that, Chuck had developed what is called a non-alcoholic fatty liver. As evidenced by his lipid panel, his cholesterol and triglycerides were significantly elevated. In addition, his fasting blood sugar was also elevated and he was slipping into type II diabetes. He felt that he had lost complete control over his health.

Chuck had been following The Plourdé Institute on social media. He was perplexed at how older, less fit men were having shocking success. This was a defining moment for Chuck, which spurred him to reach out on that fateful Monday. During his phone intake, he asked me, "Do you work with guys like me?"

I said, "Of course I do."

As an out-of-state client, he planned a trip to Chicago and went through a half-day science-based weight loss assessment.

Much to his surprise, he was given an exercise prescription of walking at 2.4 mph at an incline of approximately 12 percent. Now, this exercise prescription has been modified over time, but it was a dramatic departure from his extreme training. I instructed him not to lift weights until he plateaued, because we wanted his muscles to utilize exclusively fat and to avoid sugar cravings.

Although he heard the words that I had spoken and understood them mentally, the progress that followed shocked him to the core. The outcome that he had so painfully pursued with over-exercise came to him with ease with THE PLOURDE METHOD℠.

I remember the day of his assessment when he asked, with tears in his eyes, "How could I have not known these things?"

I said to him, "I have studied my entire life in a laboratory setting to learn these principles. Of course you couldn't have known them. Don't beat yourself up. You know them now and you're going to get everything I say, when I say, and how I say—except it's probably going to be even better."

In four months, Chuck lost over 70 percent of his body fat and he was shocked to be at 10 percent body fat at the age of sixty. Much to his surprise, after losing such a significant amount of body fat (most of this fat loss occurred from the intra-abdominal cavity), his liver function and lipid panel showed dramatic improvement: normalizing cholesterol, triglycerides, and fasting glucose. ▶▶▶

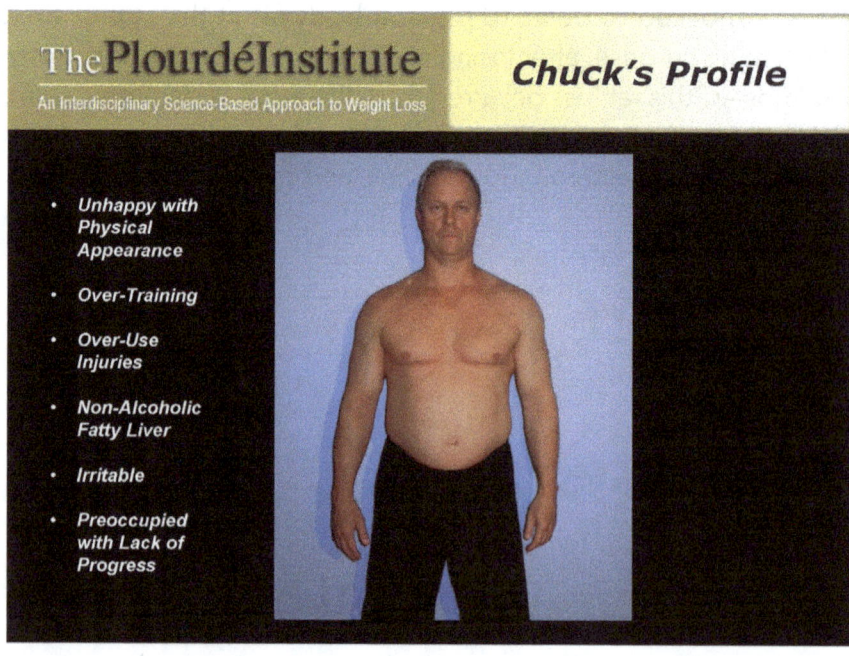

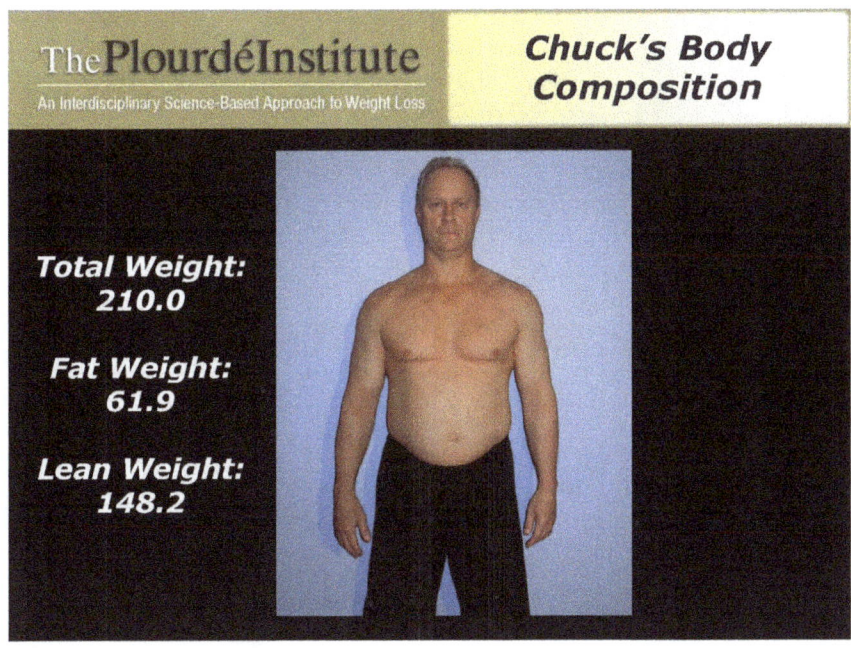

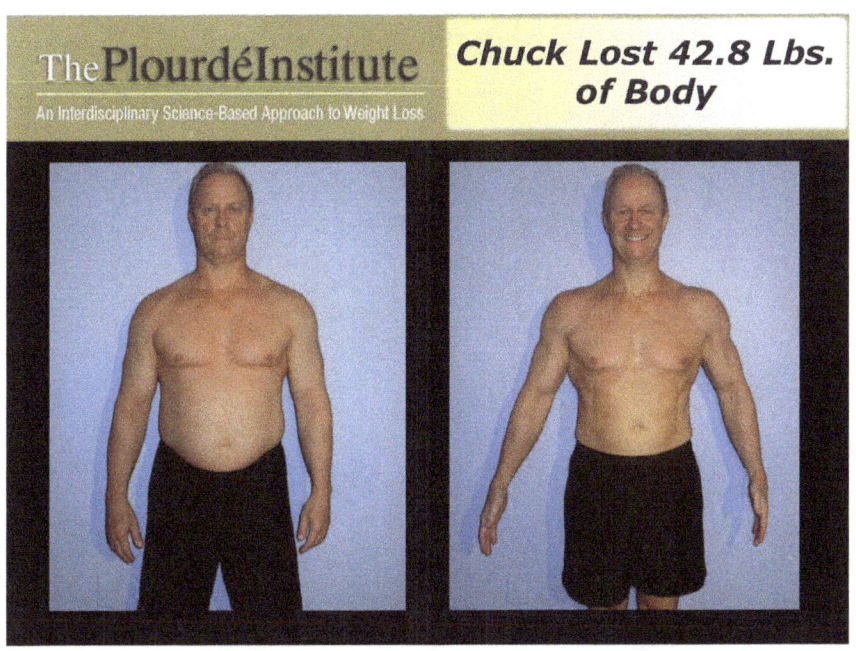

The Plourdé Institute
An Interdisciplinary Science-Based Approach to Weight Loss

Historical Evaluation of Adiposity

Name ____Chuck____ Date ___5/18/2021___

Condition of Adiposity	Baseline	Peak	Current	Goal - 50%	Goal - 60%	Goal - 71%	Goal - 75%	Goal - 80%
Body Fat %	12.0	32.0	29.5	18.8	15.4	11.5	10.0	8.2
Fat Weight	22.2	69.8	61.9	34.9	27.9	20.2	17.5	14.0
Lean Weight	162.8	148.2	148.2	150.9	153.6	156.3	156.3	156.3
Total Weight	185.0	218.0	210.1	185.8	181.5	176.5	173.8	170.3
Age	18	57	58	58	58	58	58	58
# of Adipocytes	16.8	26.4	26.4	26.4	26.4	26.4	26.4	26.4

Fat Weight Increase of ___47.6___ lbs. = ___214.4___ %

Type of Lipogenesis =

(Type 1) Adipocyte Hypertrophy ☐

(Type 2) Adipocyte Hyperplastic Hypertrophy (Both Types) ☐

Fat Weight Reduction Goal: 27.0 lbs = 43.6 %
　　　　　　　　　　　　　　34.0 lbs = 54.9 %
　　　　　　　　　　　　　　41.7 lbs = 67.3 %
　　　　　　　　　　　　　　44.5 lbs = 71.8 %
　　　　　　　　　　　　　　47.9 lbs = 77.4 %

Estimated Range of Reduction Phase = __7-9__ months

Copyright © 2023 David Plourdé, Ph.D.

The Plourdé Institute
An Interdisciplinary Science-Based Approach to Weight Loss

BODY COMPOSITION PROGRESS CHART							
CLIENT NAME: CHUCK M				GOAL FAT WEIGHT: 19.0			
DATE	TOTAL WEIGHT	FAT WEIGHT	LEAN WEIGHT	FAT LOSS	% FAT LOSS	TOTAL FAT LOSS	
5/18/2020	218.0	69.8	148.2				
5/18/2021	210.1	61.9	148.2	7.93	-11.3%	7.93	
6/12/2021	194.8	45.5	149.3	16.39	-26.5%	24.32	
7/24/2021	183.6	29.4	154.2	16.12	-35.4%	40.44	
8/28/2021	180.4	24.1	156.3	5.30	-18.0%	45.74	
10/16/2021	183.0	25.4	157.5	-1.33	+5.5%	44.41	
1/22/2022	177.4	19.1	158.3	6.33	-24.9%	50.74	

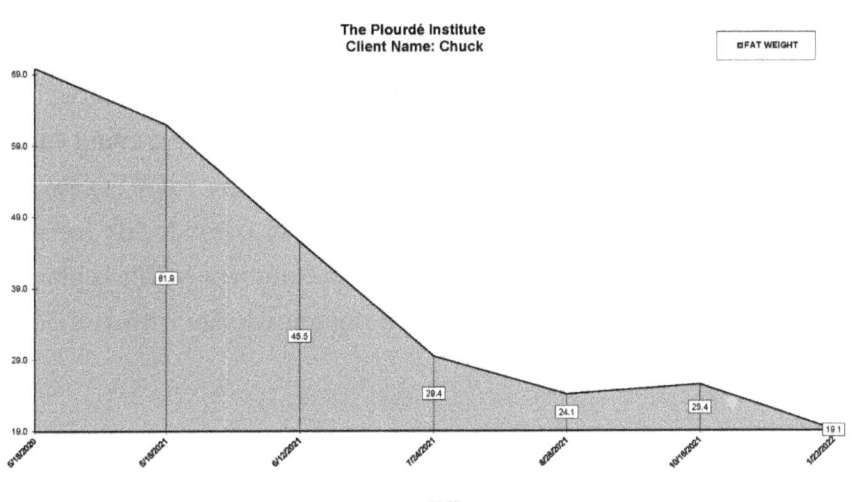

Scan the QR code to hear Chuck's amazing story:

Concluding Thought Regarding Exercise: Could Less Be More?

Do you see yourself in Scott or Chuck's story? Could it be that over-exercise has been one of the main reasons that you have not succeeded in weight loss? The answer might be yes. If you carefully apply the principles that I have outlined so far, you can expect to lose body fat weight safely and substantially without craving sugar or starches. I know that you are, in effect, hearing what I'm saying right now, but in short order these ideas will come to life for you. Although you are not in our laboratory setting where this is plainly visible, I'm so glad that I get to share my knowledge with you now!

The Plourdé Institute
An Interdisciplinary Science-Based Approach to Weight Loss

Treadmill Exercise Prescription

Name of Client _____Example_____

Time of day	First thing in the morning in a fasting state
Exercise Modality	Treadmill
Exercise Frequency	Daily
Exercise Duration	30-60 Continuous Minutes
Speed	1.8-2.6 Mph
Incline	0-15%
Heart Rate	varies
Rate of Perceived Exertion	12 Fairly Light

BORG SCALE
PERCEIVED EXERTION

6	
7	VERY, VERY LIGHT
8	
9	VERY LIGHT
10	
11	FAIRLY LIGHT
12	
13	SOMEWHAT HARD
14	
15	HARD
16	
17	VERY HARD
18	
19	VERY, VERY HARD

If you have any injuries, a hip or knee replacement, high blood pressure or any underlying cardiovascular condition, seek the advice of your medical doctor before beginning a new exercise regimen.

Copyright © 2023 David Plourdé, Ph.D.

CHAPTER 10

The Dark Side of Semaglutide Medications

In case you haven't heard, Ozempic has become a very recent weight loss craze. Unless you live off the grid, you probably already know this. The fact is, millions of people worldwide are taking semaglutide medications such as Ozempic, Wegovy, and Trulicity, just to name a few.

These medications were developed initially for the treatment of type II diabetes, and are known as glucagon inhibitors. Glucagon is a hormone that is secreted (or released) by the pancreas and increases blood sugar by signaling the liver to mobilize glucose (a process called glycogenolysis). In other words, glucagon is a hormone that raises blood sugar. By inhibiting glucagon, the liver does not release glucose and therefore helps the type II diabetic have better control of their blood sugar. It was observed that people taking semaglutide medicines also experienced weight reduction. Eventually, the FDA approved some of these diabetes medications for weight loss.

How it Works

The side effects of semaglutide seem to aid in weight loss because they slow the digestive system. First, they delay the emptying of the stomach. This was documented in the study, "Semaglutide delays four-hour gastric emptying in women with polycystic ovary syndrome and obesity" (Jensterle M, 2023). Let's continue with the explanation of how the medication works.

When the stomach remains full (gastric distention) for longer periods, the vagus nerve, which recognizes that the stomach is full, activates the satiety center of the hypothalamus (the part of the brain that tells you you're satisfied). In doing so, the part of the brain, also located in the hypothalamus, which directs what you're hungry for, how often you're hungry, and the degree of hunger (the feeding centers) *are nullified*. In application, people can have dramatic reductions in overall food intake, portions, and calories without having hunger or food cravings. This has become very appealing for those who have failed in their previous weight loss efforts.

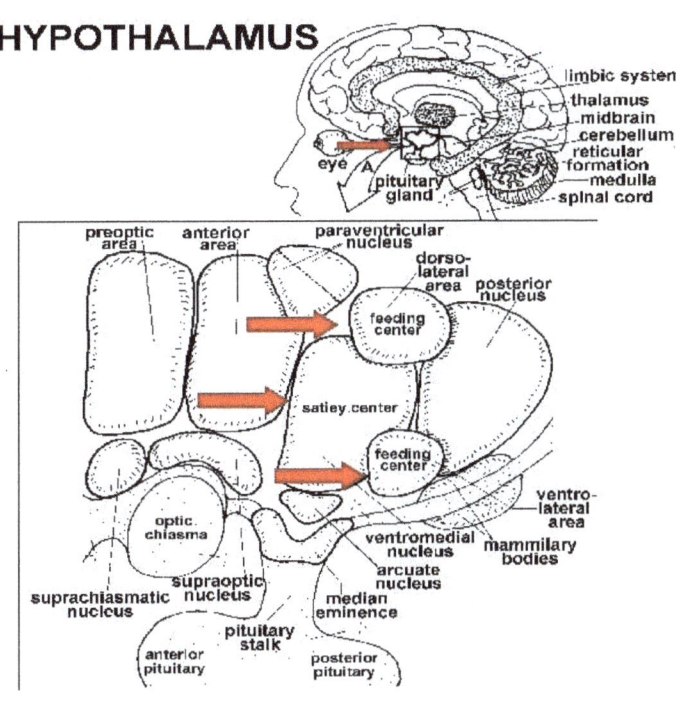

Source: (Kapit, Macey and Meisami, 1987)

Here's where the potential problems can come in ... For reasons not completely understood yet, it appears that some people have a hypersensitivity to this medication and the delayed stomach emptying may result in a halting of normal peristaltic muscle contractions (the process of ingested foods moving properly through the intestines). These conditions, termed stomach paralysis (the technical term is gastroparesis) and/or bowel obstruction, are two very serious health complications that require immediate medical intervention. Other complications can include bowel perforation (a tear in the wall of the small intestine), gallbladder disease, pancreatitis, and in some rare cases even death.

Based upon an analysis of five commonly prescribed semaglutide medicines (there are other medications that are not included in this analysis), you can see for yourself in the "Cases by Reaction" chart that I am including from the Federal Drug Administration's Adverse Events Reporting System (FAERS) the exact frequency of the top thirty-four adverse events reported. The list is so extensive I chose to limit it.

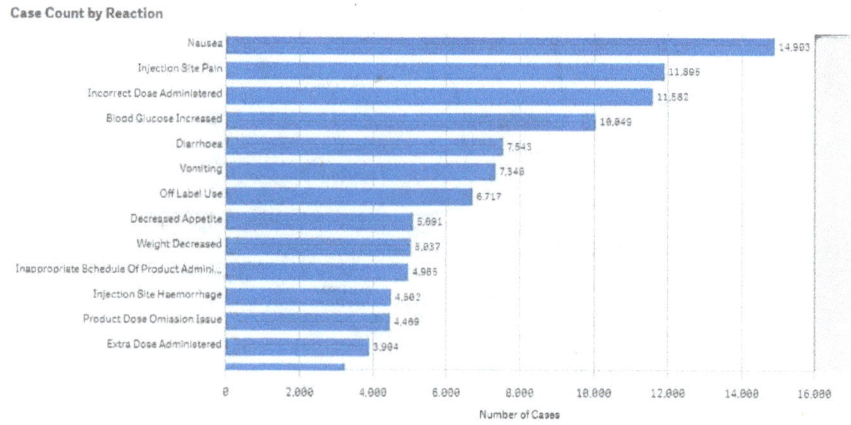

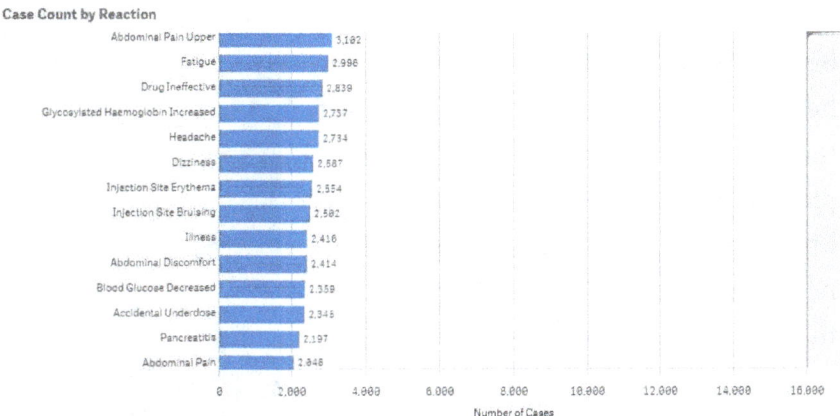

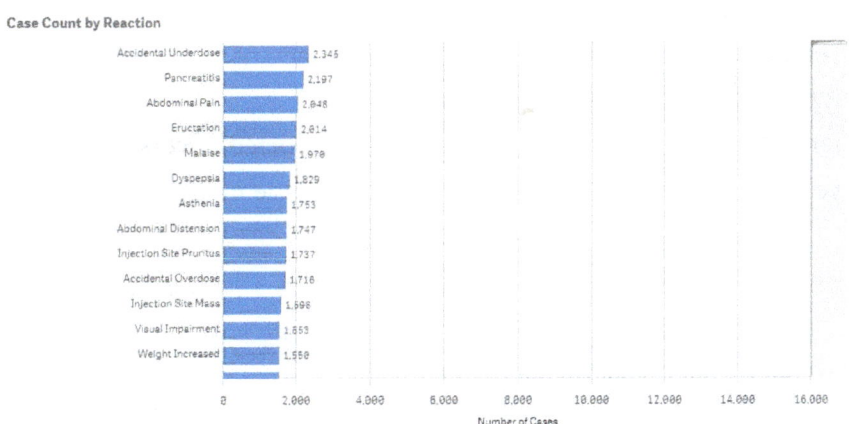

Source: FAERS website (https://fis.fda.gov 2023)

Let's take a look at a real-life example. It was reported in *The New York Post* in late 2023 that Trish Webster, a fifty-six-year-old Australian woman, died after taking Ozempic in order to lose weight for her daughter's upcoming wedding. Her husband, Roy, found her lying on the floor in the bathroom, unresponsive, with a brown liquid escaping from her mouth. She died later that night due to complications from bowel obstruction. Facing this tragic loss, he made a statement in his interview that the benefits of the weight loss drug Ozempic were not worth it, and that if they had known the risks associated, she would never have been on it. It needs to be noted that this was a rare occurrence, but a tragic one, nonetheless.

As of February 2024, the FAERS website reported 36,996 cases of adverse events in 2023 alone (for five commonly prescribed semaglutide medicines). Five of the top fifteen were gastrointestinal related problems. See FAERS data here for the total reported adverse events by year for the five most widely-used semaglutide medications:

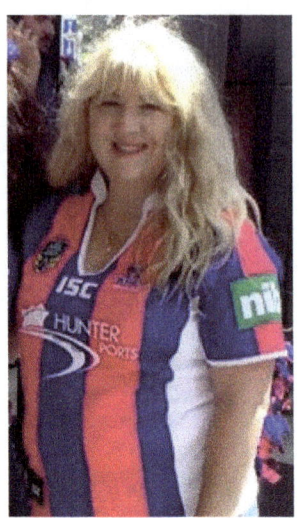

Source: Webster family photo. Used with permission

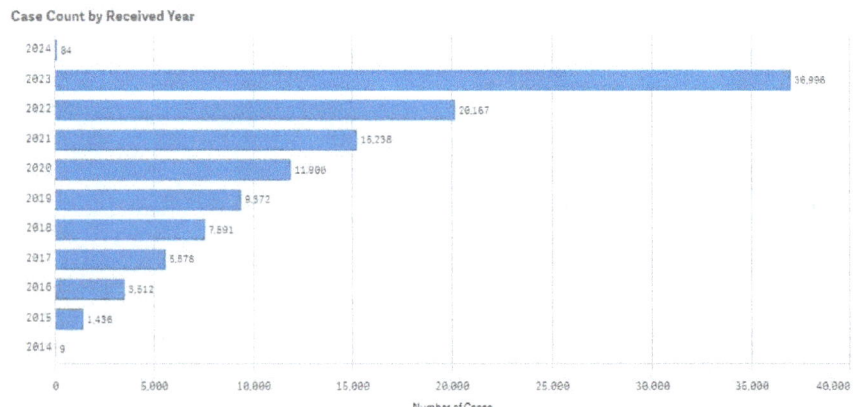

Source
Credit: FAERS Adverse Events Reporting System (FAERS) Public Dashboard (http://fis.fda.gov 2023)

Unfortunately, many people taking these medicines are accessing them by obtaining a prescription online and administering them with uneven or no real medical supervision. This is a mistake. Let me make it clear that although I'm including this chapter in my book, I'm in no way recommending these glucagon inhibitors as a weight loss intervention. But I would be intellectually dishonest if I didn't admit that they are effective for short-term weight loss—because they are.

Let's review the list of potential adverse side effects of semaglutide medications. We've already discussed stomach paralysis and bowel obstruction. Another side effect previously mentioned is gallbladder disease. Because these medicines slow the digestive system, bile salts (a digestive compound to aid in the chemical digestion of fat) are manufactured in the liver and delivered to the gallbladder through a tube called the bile duct. If bile salts sit too long in the gallbladder, they become susceptible to the formation of clusters called gallstones. If the gallstones are larger than the sphincter (the valve that ultimately opens to disperse bile salt), it can result in abdominal pain and inflammation of the gallbladder. If not treated promptly, this can result in an infection and can be potentially very dangerous. Similarly, the same medications can cause pancreatitis for the following reasons: if a gallstone occludes the path of both bile salt and digestive enzymes coming from the pancreas at the location of the common duct, the interruption of these digestive properties can cause inflammation of the pancreas (a vital organ of the human body).

Another observation of the risks associated with semaglutide is lung aspiration during surgical procedures. If you've ever had surgery, you know that the medical staff will instruct you to refrain from eating after dinner the night before your procedure. Under normal conditions, this allows the stomach to have the appropriate amount of time to properly empty itself into the small intestine. However, because glucagon inhibitors delay the emptying of the stomach, undigested food contents, in some cases, have backed up into the lungs causing aspiration and death. Therefore, some anesthesiologists are suggesting that patients should have much more time off of the medication prior to surgery to prevent this potentially life-threatening circumstance.

Here you will see a diagram of the digestive system and where these problems can occur. Let me remind you that I am not a medical doctor, and if you suffer these symptoms, you need to contact your primary care physician right away. This needs to be taken seriously. I am in no way suggesting that this chapter be taken as medical advice. Your safety is my highest priority. My scientific credentials are in human nutrition and exercise physiology—not medicine.

Let me also point out that there's no data available on the long-term use of semaglutide medicines for non-type II diabetics. Could there be other risks associated with long term use of these medications? Only time will tell.

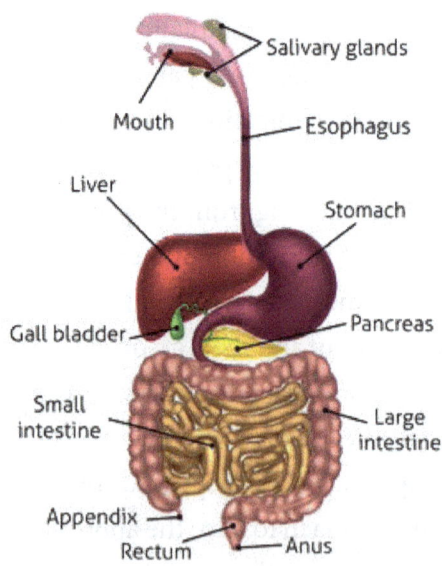

Source: Development of Foregut by Neeta Chhabra (Chhabra, 2020)

The other big question is if the use of glucagon inhibitors will eventually need to be discontinued for the non-type II diabetic. If and when the medicine is discontinued, normal hypothalamic directed hunger will resume. In some cases, people may experience 'boomerang hunger', which is a cycle of hunger that cannot be predicted, controlled, or satisfied until fat cell weight and body fat weight return to previous levels.

In some ways, the semaglutide medicines may be an appealing biohack. However, all of the other necessary puzzle pieces are missing: nutrition, exercise physiology, psychology of eating behavior, food addiction recovery, as well as appropriate accountability. Absent of these necessary pieces, regaining whatever initial weight loss was experienced is almost a certainty.

Something else you should be aware of is that not all weight loss is equal. When calorie restriction is the sole modality in a weight loss effort, as it is with these medications and gastric bypass, nearly one-third of weight loss comes from valuable lean tissue (muscles, bones, connective tissues, and organs). This was clearly documented in the published paper entitled "Bioexponential Model for Predicting Weight-Loss after Gastric Surgery for Obesity" (Livingston, 2001) that examined a small group (twenty-eight obese adult human subjects, prescreened for psychological and emotional readiness for treatment) who underwent gastric bypass. All participants were subjected to body composition testing to assess changes in body fat and lean tissue. The average body fat loss for the subjects was approximately 73 percent. But the alarming finding was that approximately **27 percent of their total weight loss came from lean tissue.** Although Ozempic and medicines like it are different from a gastric bypass procedure, the weight loss occurs for similar reasons: calorie reduction, portion control, and enhanced satiety, as well as other factors that we are not aware of yet.

In the case of semaglutide, the feeding centers are nullified or inhibited because of the slowing of the digestive system, whereas with gastric bypass, enhanced satiety is achieved because of a surgical resizing of the stomach. So, although no scientific journal articles have been published yet (that I am aware of) related to body composition changes associated with glucagon inhibitors, it is reasonable to expect that the metabolic implications of such an intervention would have a similar effect on the make-up of fat and lean tissue. This might be an area for future research.

You might be asking yourself, "How can there be such a dramatic loss of lean tissue with certain weight loss interventions?"

Here's how. Under normal metabolic conditions, when you're eating, *not fasting*, cellular respiration (the technical term for metabolism) has essentially two options:

First, the body can utilize fatty acids (fat), which come from the broken triglycerides and subsequently mobilized fatty acids from your fat cells. This metabolic pathway is called oxidative phosphorylation. In layman's terms: this means the cells can use fat as a fuel source in cellular work *as long as oxygen is present in the cell.*

The **second** option for fuel consumption in cellular respiration is the utilization of glucose (sugar). This metabolic process occurs in the absence of oxygen in the cell and is called anaerobic glycolysis.

However, there is a **third** option for fuel utilization in the cell that occurs specifically in a fasting state, and it's called gluconeogenesis. It's a technical term, but it essentially means that the body can convert proteins, called amino acids, coming from muscles and organs into energy. Let me make clear that this is a metabolic adaptation that occurs when the body is in *crisis*, and it becomes very evident in conditions such as anorexia or bulimia. It is also observed in circumstances of starvation when the body uniquely catabolizes (breaks down and utilizes) valuable lean tissues for survival.

I think you get the picture at this point, don't you? The semaglutide medicines work, but not without some undesirable outcomes and potential dangers. There may be other approaches that are just as effective, if not more effective, without the potential risks. At the end of the day, your weight loss journey is your decision, but in my professional opinion, these medicines are not an option that I would recommend.

Subsection: THE PLOURDE METHOD℠— A Healthy Alternative to Semaglutide Medications

Consider this scenario: You tried a semaglutide medicine and in short order felt symptoms of nausea and perhaps other gastrointestinal symptoms to such a degree that you knew you couldn't continue to take it. As a result, you're having deep feelings of despair with no way forward to solve your problem with unsuccessful weight loss.

Or here's another scenario you might be facing: You know several people that are taking these medicines and they are having successful weight loss, but after reading certain articles or seeing news segments about these medicines and their associated risks, you've decided that it's not worth it.

Here's another possible circumstance: You've started the semaglutide medicine for the sole purpose of losing weight and you are not a type II diabetic. In your gut you know that at some point you will have to discontinue the medicine. All the benefits of negating hunger will dissipate and you'll inevitably be back to square one, facing a tidal wave of hunger that you can't predict, control, or satisfy.

Any way we slice it, you feel discouraged and without hope. Well, I have good news for you . . .

Let me give you several reasons why THE PLOURDE METHOD℠ can be a healthy alternative to semaglutide medications:

1. When you include low to moderate protein at breakfast, lunch, and dinner, it prolongs the time of chemical digestion in the small intestine, subsequently slowing the rate of absorption of all nutrients into the blood stream. This has a steadying effect on blood sugar, which results in reduced insulin production,

lengthened satiety periods, and the absence of hunger. The protein portions are specifically low to moderate, *not* high, because too much protein will constipate you, ultimately creating circumstances similar to the adverse events associated with semaglutide. So please review the meal plan chapter and apply the appropriate protein portions, being careful not to exceed them.

2. When following a moderate fat diet, stomach emptying is delayed. For the same reason previously mentioned above, the satiety centers remain activated and therefore the feeding centers are nullified. You will not be hungry and will very likely not have cravings. Be careful, though. Too much fat will result in excessive acid production (in an effort of predigestion) and can lead to acid reflux, nausea, and indigestion—not fun. So, to be clear, the recommended regimen is neither low fat, because that would result in a rapid emptying of the stomach, triggering sudden hunger; nor is it high fat, which triggers acid indigestion. A moderate fat diet is spelled out very clearly in the meal plan section. So please revisit that chapter and be careful to maintain the appropriate fat sources and subsequent portions.

3. Half of the dietary regimen comes from high-fiber, non-sugar, non-starch vegetables. For some of you, this will mean you're eating more vegetables now than you've ever eaten in your life. Vegetables such as raw or lightly cooked broccoli or cauliflower (with the stem) and celery have more complex chemical composition and will pass through the small intestine with minimal chemical digestion. The vast majority of their content will move into the large intestine, where the body absorbs water and minerals through the walls of the

large intestine into the bloodstream. Because these vegetables are bulky and contain significant amounts of water, more significant gastric distention (or stomach filling) will occur. This will produce a prolonged satiety period, nullifying the feeding centers of the hypothalamus. As a result, you won't be hungry, and you will likely not have food cravings.

4. A very important point to remember is that for many people when they think about what it means to be 'on plan,' their thoughts are focused on their selections of food and fluid. Inherently, they believe that if their choices are in alignment with the METHOD, they are fully 'on plan.' However, that is not accurate, because 50 percent of what it means to be on program has to do with eating behavior. I teach my clients to eat on an interval of every two and a half hours whether hungry or not. This may feel strange to you because you're eating prior to getting hungry. The major benefit in doing so is that the feeding centers never have a chance to activate and therefore prolong the satiety period. This is the main reason why the semaglutide medicines have become so popular. This is another section you can review in the meal plan chapter.

In summary, the regimen outlined in this book will allow you to experience significant body fat weight loss while sparing valuable lean tissue without the potential risks of semaglutide medicines. Does that sound like a good plan to you?

CHAPTER 11

Are You Ready to Be Accountable?

Accountability is a NON-NEGOTIATABLE piece of your weight loss puzzle. The business guru, David Drucker, has been quoted as saying, "What gets measured gets managed." Another version of this quote is, "What gets measured gets done." It's up for debate who originally coined these phrases, so I'll leave it at that.

Although accountability has not really been mentioned until this moment, the principle of accountability has been present in every client success story. First of all, what does the word accountability actually mean? It comes from the root word account, which means "a statement explaining one's conduct"(*Merriam-Webster*). From a business / financial perspective, to account is "a statement of transactions during a fiscal period and the resulting balance" (*Merriam-Webster*). Accountability is defined in the dictionary as "the fact of being responsible for what you do and able to give a satisfactory reason for it, or the degree to which this happens" (*Cambridge Business English Dictionary* website).

In the context of weight loss, I have defined accountability as one's willingness to record precisely what you eat, what you drink, how you eat and drink, as well as details of your sleep patterns, energy levels, stress, bowel movements, and exercise. When I conducted my original research, all of the subjects were required to log these factors, check in daily via phone or daily text, and show up for weekly in-laboratory assessments. Anyone that was not willing to fully cooperate in this manner was excluded from the study.

I was particularly interested in what would happen with compliant subjects. Not to be negative, but we all know what happens with non-compliance: failure. You are here right now reading this book. You took a risk and made the sacrifice to buy this book for a reason: to replace your pain with a life of better health, joy, and self-respect. If that's true, GO NO FURTHER until you internalize this idea.

I want to again thank every person who unselfishly and generously shared their story. Each of these individuals made an unequivocal decision to be accountable. And, if you want to succeed in your own weight loss journey, you also will need to make a *real* decision. The word decision comes from the root word scission, which means, "to cut." De-cision means, "to cut off from all other options in a specific course of action." It means you're going to leave yourself no other option but to move forward.

As uncomfortable as facing our psychological and emotional pains may be, it is our pain that can help us get out of our comfort zone and take the necessary action that we need to take.

I think we can all agree that being accountable requires discipline. If you've lacked discipline in your life, especially in this area, this is where we go no further until you fully digest the message of this chapter. Are you ready to be accountable?

If you can relate to the main character of the story: a person who's winning in pretty much every area of life except one, you're overweight, and you're not recording what you eat, what you drink, how you eat and drink, as well as the other factors mentioned above, you can forget about any substantial weight loss success.

You may have heard the phrase "perception is not reality." I've observed for many years that people often do not actually know what they're eating and drinking. They think they know, but the truth is they often are completely disconnected and it's this lack of personal awareness that keeps people from getting substantial traction in their weight loss efforts.

Furthermore, the subject of being overweight can cause immense pain for people: shame, embarrassment, self-loathing, anger, isolation, fear, anxiety—it can be very dark. As intimidating as accountability can be, it's instrumental for us to move forward into a better quality of life. When people get stuck in a rut and fall off track in their weight loss journey, I've noticed a common pattern: people may engage in avoidance behavior. They will cancel their appointments at the last second with the most creative excuses, but the tendency is undeniable: people don't like to be accountable when they feel embarrassed or ashamed. Oftentimes, our biggest obstacle in our forward path is ourselves. Being accountable doesn't mean that you have to be perfect, but it does require a certain modicum of humility and receptivity. This is not weakness. On the contrary, these are admirable traits commonly found in successful people.

Many people who have tried weight loss apps or engaged in online weight loss experiences have had some progress, but others have found these approaches to be unsuccessful. One of the missing pieces in these approaches may be the lack of *real* accountability. Accountability does not occur between your ears, with a bot, or with AI; it happens in a relationship with another human being.

I have observed for years that people that are accountable in their weight loss journey are far more successful than those who are not. In Alcoholics Anonymous® (AA) there is a phrase that says, "we are only as sick as our secrets." In the Bible, in the book of James, it says, "Therefore confess your sins to each other and pray for each other so that you may be healed. The prayer of a righteous person is powerful and effective" (James 5:16 NIV).

I'm not suggesting that eating unhealthy food is immoral, what I'm saying here is that when two people are transparent and sincerely open with each other, it results in a deep healing. For most of us, when we feel like we're "off the rails" with our so-called diet, we can feel angry, ashamed, and frustrated with ourselves. This often leads to the avoidance behavior previously mentioned.

It's been observed for decades in AA that when somebody "falls off the wagon," they often don't get back on the wagon until they get to their next meeting. This is a profound truth, and there is remarkable similarity in the weight loss process. Let me insert a very important point here. When you feel these dark emotions because your eating behavior is entirely incongruent with your health and fitness goals; when every fiber of your being wants to cancel your appointment with your trainer, weight loss coach, therapist, or physician—DON'T DO IT! Resist these self-sabotaging tendencies. Be open and honest with your accountability person and anticipate a reversal of your circumstances. I know this may be hard for you to believe, but I've been witnessing this profound truth for many years. Therefore, **BE ACCOUNTABLE. The Three Essential Pieces for Effective Weight Loss Accountability**

1. **Log** food and fluid selections, eating and drinking behaviors, exercise, sleep, stress, bowel movements (evacuations), and emotional inventory.
2. **Have a brief daily touchpoint** with your chosen accountability partner to ensure you're staying on track.

3. **Show up** for weekly (ideally in-person) progress reviews with your chosen coach.

To demonstrate the power of accountability in the weight loss journey, let me share with you the following client case study:

▶▶▶ Agnes arrived at The Plourdé Institute for a weight loss assessment on Tuesday, November 4, 2014. She was fifty-five years old and a leader in a Fortune 500 company. She was 5'4" tall and was just shy of 190 pounds. Agnes was happily married and succeeding in every area of her life except that she was overweight. In fact, she could not have been more uncomfortable, unhappy, or dissatisfied with her physical appearance. Her weight was an impending distraction. We placed Agnes in the BOD POD on that fateful day and learned that of the 189.7 pounds of total weight, 87.4 pounds was lean tissue and 102.2 pounds was body fat. This was her all-time highest body fat level.

We continued the assessment and conducted several other lab measurements: a VO2 max stress test as well as metabolic measurement testing. We went on to forecast her body fat weight loss journey that would ultimately land somewhere between 61 and 73 percent body fat weight loss from her present/peak fat weight. Taking in all of the information, she thoughtfully but decisively moved forward with the program.

We conducted body composition measurements in the BOD POD every four weeks. As you can plainly see from her spreadsheets, her body fat weight loss ranged from 11 to 16 percent per month every month until a plateau formed. Her body fat weight went from 102.2 to 28.8 pounds, representing a 73.5 pound body fat weight loss. In addition, she gained six pounds of muscle. She could not have been more thrilled.

Agnes points out in her testimonial video that having someone who was not just a doctor, but also a mentor and accountability person, made a huge impact on her success story. She specifically mentions that having a coach that was unconditionally supportive and non-judgmental created a sense of safety. She never felt like she was going to get scolded if she went off the meal plan. As a result, she always showed up to her appointments and maintained a positive attitude.

Her accountability structure included logging her foods daily and journaling, engaging with daily text messages, and showing up for weekly sessions in the laboratory to measure the cumulative impact of her overall program compliance throughout the week. She spoke about the importance of daily text messages. Knowing she would receive a text every day asking about how she was doing helped her to stay on track and forge through the difficult periods where in the past she would've fallen off track.

Recalling the quote from the beginning of the chapter, "What gets measured gets managed" we can see clearly, Agnes benefited from consistent objective measurements, accountability, and encouragement. It helped her to stay on track throughout her journey. See her before and after pictures as well as her spreadsheets in the pages ahead: ▶▶▶

Are You Ready to Be Accountable? 145

The Plourdé Institute
An Interdisciplinary Science-Based Approach to Weight Loss

BODY COMPOSITION PROGRESS CHART							
CLIENT NAME: AGNES				GOAL FAT WEIGHT: 35.5			
DATE	TOTAL WEIGHT	FAT WEIGHT	LEAN WEIGHT	FAT LOSS	% FAT LOSS	TOTAL FAT LOSS	
11/4/2014	189.7	102.2	87.4				
12/3/2014	175.2	87.0	88.2	15.24	-14.9%	15.24	
1/7/2015	163.6	74.8	88.8	12.17	-14.0%	27.41	
2/4/2015	155.8	66.5	89.3	8.33	-11.1%	35.74	
3/6/2015	147.7	58.8	88.9	7.70	-11.6%	43.44	
4/8/2015	139.1	48.9	90.2	9.90	-16.8%	53.34	
5/6/2015	134.9	43.5	91.4	5.37	-11.0%	58.71	
6/3/2015	130.1	38.1	92.0	5.45	-12.5%	64.16	
7/8/2015	127.6	34.6	93.0	3.44	-9.0%	67.60	
8/5/2015	122.3	28.8	93.5	5.86	-16.9%	73.46	
9/15/2015	125.7	32.2	93.5	-3.37	+11.7%	70.08	
10/13/2015	126.4	33.0	93.5	-0.80	+2.5%	69.28	
11/17/2015	125.1	31.8	93.3	1.18	-3.6%	70.46	
1/5/2016	127.6	35.6	92.0	-3.86	+12.2%	66.60	

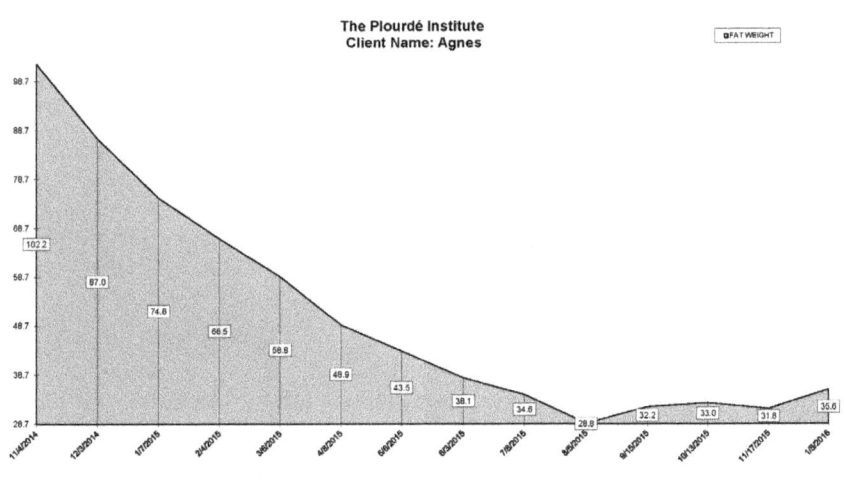

The Plourdé Institute
An Interdisciplinary Science-Based Approach to Weight Loss

Historical Evaluation of Adiposity

Name _____Agnes_____ Date _____11/04/2014_____

Condition of Adiposity	Baseline	Peak/ Current	Goal -50%	Goal -60%	Goal -65%	Goal -70%
Body Fat %	20.0	53.9	36.7	31.5	28.5	25.3
Fat Weight	23.0	102.2	51.1	40.9	35.8	30.7
Lean Weight	92.0	87.4	88.2	88.9	89.7	90.4
Total Weight	115.0	189.7	139.3	129.8	125.4	121.0
Age	16	55	55	55	55	55
# of Adipocytes (in Billions)	17.4	38.6	38.6	38.6	38.6	38.6

Fat Weight Increase of __79.2__ lbs. = __344.5__ %

Type of Lipogenesis =

(Type 1) Adipocyte Hypertrophy ☐

(Type 2) Adipocyte Hyperplastic Hypertrophy (Both Types) ☐

Fat Weight Reduction Goal: 51.1 lbs = 50.0 %
  61.3 lbs = 60.0 %
  66.4 lbs = 65.0 %
  71.6 lbs = 70.0 %

Estimated Range of Reduction Phase = __9__ months

Copyright © 2023 David Plourdé

Are You Ready to Be Accountable? 147

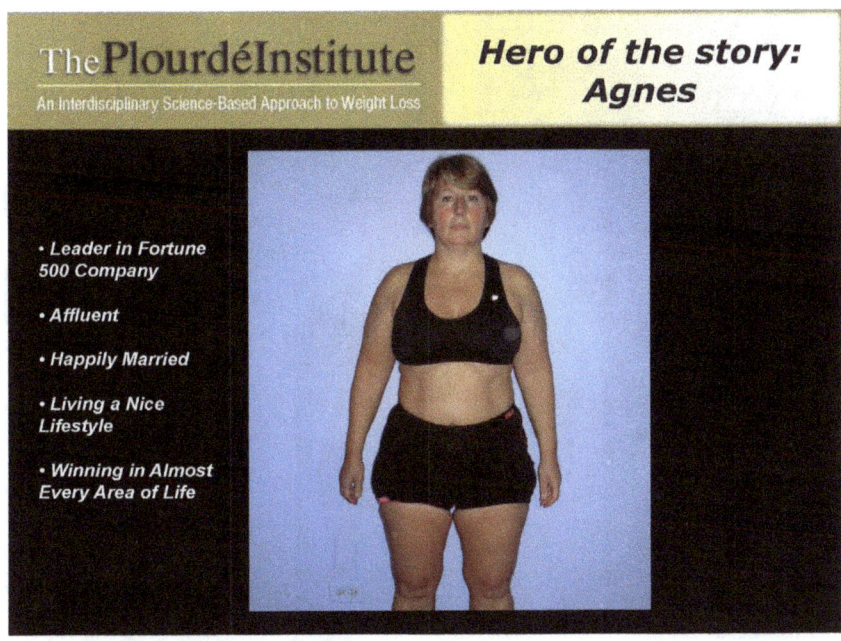

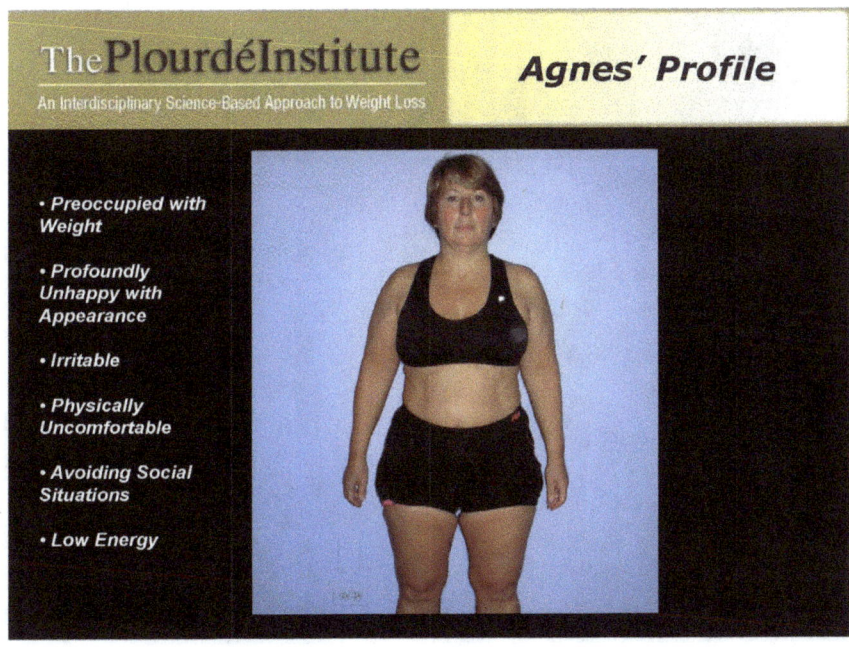

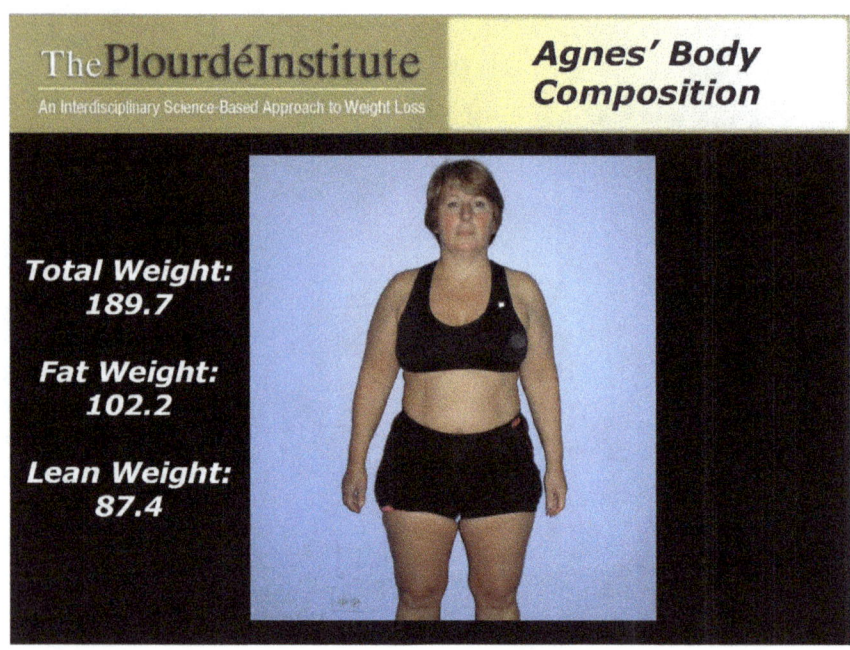

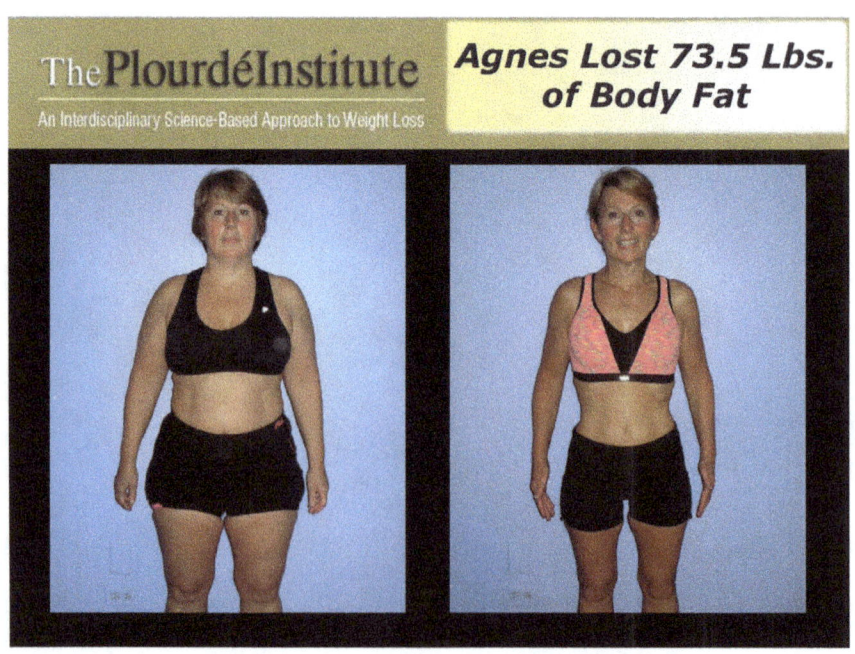

Scan the QR code to hear Agnes tell her story:

Could accountability be a missing piece for you? Let's remedy that and get you moving in the right direction. I will share some accountability resources that may be helpful to you in the Personal Invitation chapter.

Chapter 12
Your Body Fat, Your Health, and Disease

If you're middle-aged or older, overweight, and have been working with a medical doctor over the course of your life, you may have noticed that your cholesterol levels, your triglyceride levels, and your fasting blood glucose are all elevating. Though this may not be true for everyone, this chapter will connect the dots between increasing body fat levels and disease progression. If you're confused and feeling a certain level of fear about these trends, you're not alone. These are, unfortunately, common patterns that people observe in the course of their aging process, but it doesn't have to be that way. This chapter will explain why these trends are occurring and what you can do to change them.

In my opinion, human body composition testing, as a laboratory measurement, may be the greatest single indicator of the cumulative impact that your lifestyle is having on your body, perhaps more so than any other single test. Here's why:

Body fat weight is simply the weight of all fat cells. When fat cells are extracted from a person who has a normal level of body fat and has never been overweight, each fat cell weighs approximately 0.7 of a microgram.

Your Body Fat, Your Health, and Disease   151

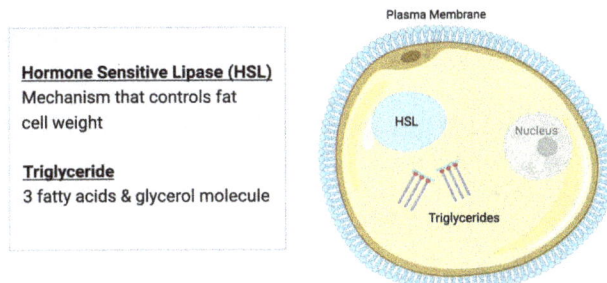

Credit: Created in BioRender. Plourde, D., Plourde, B. (2024)
BioRender.com/m65f625

Conversely, when fat cells are extracted from an obese individual who is at their highest level of body fat in their lifetime, fat cells can weigh as much as 1.4 micrograms. Did you catch that? **Fat cell weight can only double. This has a very important clinical significance.**

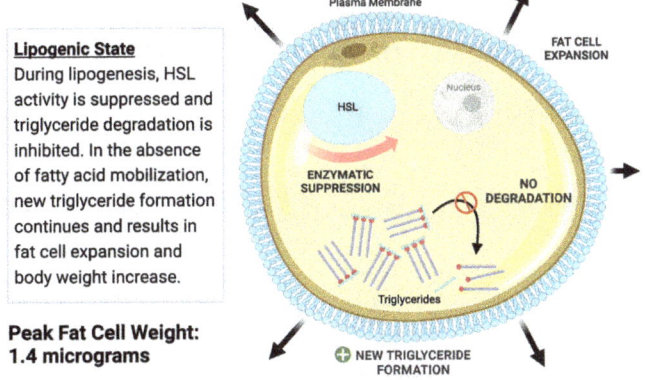

Credit: Created in BioRender. Plourde, D., Plourde, B. (2024)
BioRender.com/b68u802

When body fat weight more than doubles, it points to the fact that there are actually two types of fat creation, or lipogenesis. The first type is when fat cells get larger, it's called Adipocyte Hypertrophy.

Lipogenesis Type I:
Adipocyte Hypertrophy

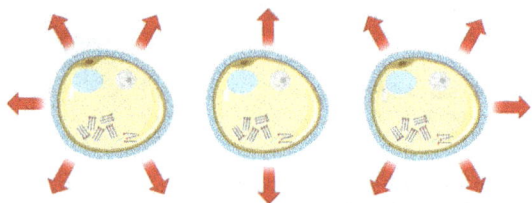

Fat cells expand and grow larger

Credit: Created in BioRender. Plourde, D., Plourde, B. (2024)
BioRender.com/j68y821

The second type is when new fat cells are manufactured in the body and it's called Adipocyte Hyperplastic Hypertrophy.

Lipogenesis Type II:
Adipocyte Hyperplastic Hypertrophy

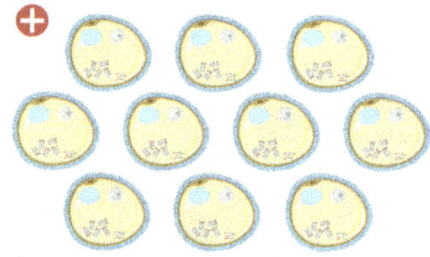

Fat cells increase in number

Credit: Created in BioRender. Plourde, D., Plourde, B. (2024)
BioRender.com/f35o957

Your Body Fat, Your Health, and Disease 153

When new fat cells are manufactured, where they are located is genetically determined. There are several patterns of type two lipogenesis. Please find the illustrations of patterns of fat distribution here:

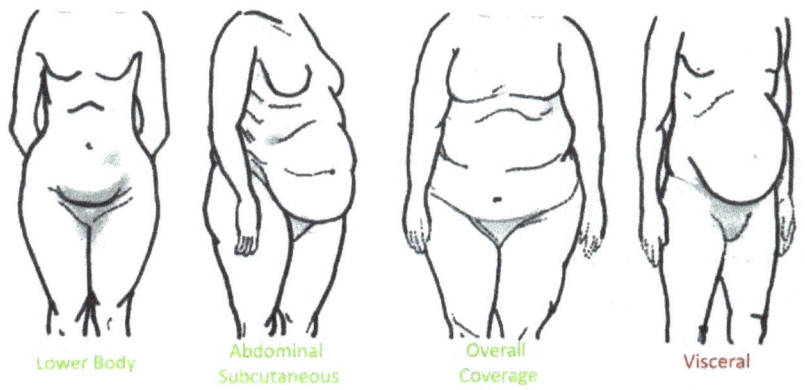

Lower Body   Abdominal Subcutaneous   Overall Coverage   Visceral

Source: (Foster, 2012)

I want to pay particular attention to the type II lipogenesis pattern, where new fat cells accumulate in the abdominal cavity. We call this intra-abdominal or visceral fat. When new fat cells accumulate in this region, they may very likely encroach the liver, leading to a condition called non-alcoholic fatty liver. This is a very serious condition. Let me explain why.

Imagine that at this moment my blood glucose levels are elevated. With a normal functioning liver, some of the excess glucose will be diverted to the liver, where it will be stored in the form of glycogen—a polymer of glucose. As a result, blood glucose levels naturally go down.

Conversely, imagine my blood glucose levels are low. With a normal functioning liver, it will conduct a process called glycogenolysis—a fancy term for breaking glycogen into pieces and subsequently, releasing glucose into the bloodstream. Naturally, blood glucose levels will rise back to normal. However, for the person who has type II lipogenesis, where the new fat cells are accumulating predominantly in the abdominal cavity, these new fat cells may encroach on the liver. When this happens, their body loses this buffer for blood glucose regulation.

Here's where things become physiologically dangerous: under these circumstances, in the absence of a normal functioning liver, the body may compensate with hyper-insulin secretion. As the liver continues to grow more fatty, the pancreas will over-secrete insulin to maintain normal glucose levels. Unfortunately, this predisposes the fat cells to a continuous state of HSL suppression, perpetually increasing body fat weight.

In addition, as fat tissue accumulates in the abdomen, it will obstruct the diaphragm (a muscle that moves the lungs up and down to help you breathe), making it difficult for the body to pull oxygen from the surrounding air through the lungs and into the blood. As a result, over time blood oxygen saturation may decrease.

For the person who suffers from this pattern of fat distribution, it means that blood pressure will slowly and continuously elevate to accelerate the uptake of oxygen from the surrounding air through the lungs and into the blood. So, not only will this individual suffer from hyper-insulin secretion, continuous fat synthesis, and inflammation, but they will also be susceptible to high blood pressure and an increased risk of heart attack and stroke. Need I mention that increased risk of sleep apnea will also accompany these conditions? Not good!

To help bring this content to life, let me introduce to you one of my star pupils: Martin.

▶▶▶ Martin was fifty-five years old when he came in for his assessment. He is the chairman of a $500 million business and was succeeding in every way possible, except his health. Besides being clinically overweight, he also suffered from a non-alcoholic fatty liver. He was working with a special physician, called a lipidologist, for over ten years. This physician's primary focus was

Your Body Fat, Your Health, and Disease 155

to help improve liver function, yet he saw no success in clearing the liver of excess fat. In addition, Martin was a type II diabetic. He was under the supervision of numerous physicians and taking statin medications to lower his cholesterol along with Metformin to control blood sugar. He coupled all of these efforts by working with a personal trainer, where he engaged in vigorous exercise several times a week. Although Martin had lost approximately twenty pounds and gained a little bit of muscle, he was unfortunately not seeing any improvement with his liver function, type II diabetes, or any of his other maladies. This was confusing, frustrating, and very discouraging for him. How could he be working so hard and being so diligent and still not get any meaningful traction?

At this point, he was referred to me by another successful client, Paul (also mentioned in Chapter 8), who had lost over fifty-two pounds of fat (70.5 percent of his total body fat weight) and gained ten pounds of muscle with THE PLOURDE METHOD℠ at the age of sixty.

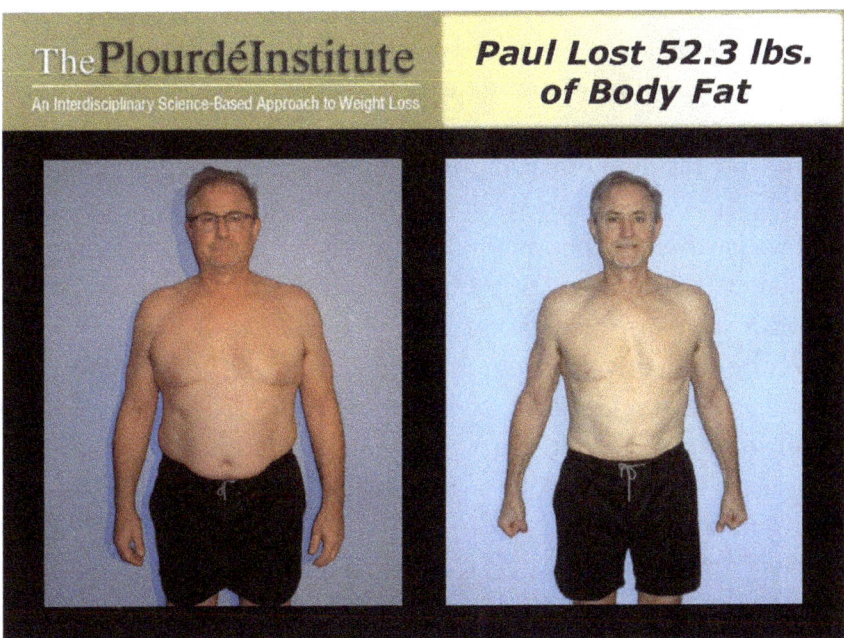

You can hear Paul's story by scanning the QR code:

Inspired by Paul, Martin came to the Institute for a weight loss assessment on February 11, 2022. What we extrapolated during the assessment is that Martin had slightly high body fat at the age of eighteen. This translated to a total body weight of 205 pounds, 36.9 pounds of body fat, 168.1 pounds of lean tissue. Fast forward to the age of forty-nine, when he then weighed 280 pounds and had 121.9 pounds of fat and ten pounds less muscle. This was his all-time highest body fat level.

On the day of the initial testing, Martin's body fat was measured in the BOD POD at 90.1 pounds, and with the help of his trainer, he had gained back the 10 pounds of muscle that he had lost. When comparing his baseline body fat at the age of eighteen to his peak body fat at the age of forty-nine, we realized he had increased his body fat weight by over eighty-five pounds, or a 230.4 percent increase in total body fat.

This is where the connection to body fat, health, and disease intersect. Remember, body fat weight is simply the weight of all your fat cells. Normal fat cells in a man or woman who has never been overweight weigh approximately 0.7 of a microgram. When you extract fat cells from a person at their highest body fat level, we have learned that the heaviest fat cells ever measured in obese human subjects is double the size of a normal fat cell at 1.4 micrograms.

Here's the connection: As I just explained, when body fat weight more than doubles, the body manufactures **new** fat cells, and where these new fat cells accumulate is genetically inherited. In the case of Martin, a substantial percentage of the new fat cells accumulated in the intra-abdominal cavity, and as a result, they encroached his liver, and he developed the condition of non-alcoholic fatty liver.

Here's an important clinical insight regarding Martin's health history: when he was eighteen years old, he had approximately 27.9 billion fat cells (which may sound like a really high fat cell number, but it is actually a relatively normal fat cell number for an eighteen-year-old male). However, after a 230.4 percent increase in body fat, we estimated that his fat cell number had climbed to 46.1 billion. A disproportionate amount of these new fat cells had accumulated in the abdomen, as I have previously mentioned. As you will soon plainly see from Martin's upper body side view photos, the predominant change in body composition occurred within the abdominal cavity.

The cumulative impact of THE PLOURDE METHOD℠ on Martin's body composition had significant positive implications regarding his lipid panel and comprehensive metabolic panel. Needless to say, Martin and his physicians were elated with this change. I'm not suggesting that the METHOD is a medical intervention—it is not. I'm simply communicating that when body fat weight reduces for a clinically overweight individual, it may have a significant impact on body systems and overall physiology.

The idea that I led with in this book regarding my early research objectives was first to develop a method to monitor HSL, later to learn how to fully control it, and finally to establish a statistical tool to predict when the body would resist further fat cell weight reduction.

The little-known fact that I want to make clear is that your adipose tissue (total body fat weight) responds in concert-like fashion, like a conductor leading an orchestra. While in suppression, fat cell weight goes up from top to bottom, and when HSL is reactivated, conversely, they all reduce.

What this means from a health perspective is that the fat cells located in the abdomen will also continuously mobilize. This means that if the body fat in the abdomen reduces, it literally shrinks, and if it remains in a continuous state of mobilization, the liver may actually clear of the fat, reversing the non-alcoholic fatty liver. See Martin's labs at 121.9 pounds of body fat compared with 24.7 pounds of body fat weight below. You can't deny it. It's remarkable!

Body Fat Weight & Blood Tests
97 lb. Fat Loss (79.6% reduction)

Body Fat Weight	Fasting Glucose	Total Cholesterol	Triglycerides
121.9 lbs	118	250	324
24.7 lbs	87	110	140

Source: The Plourdé Institute

There were signs of reversal of the non-alcoholic fatty liver after just four months. Ultimately, Martin experienced a 70 percent reduction in fat weight, and when he saw his lipidologist, all of the markers had improved. This was an astounding outcome, and it was an outcome that Martin had sought for over ten years to no avail. ▶▶▶

The important point I need to add here is that when a person has experienced a body fat weight increase of more than 100 percent and the body enters into type II fat creation, the new fat cells that are created are permanent. What does this mean?

In application, it means that for a person who has had a two-, three- or four-fold increase in fat cell number, their body will be more sensitive to the suppression caused by both obvious and insidious carbohydrates. Instead of 20 billion fat cells saying, "Gimme, gimme, gimme," you may have 30, 40, 50 billion or more fat cells saying, "Gimme, gimme, gimme."

For this individual, they will need to be more careful in their long-term diet compliance. It's the reason why after people lose weight of any significant amount, the bodies of those who have had extensive type II fat creation respond in a manner dissimilar to the person who never increased their fat cell number.

In the movie *Top Gun*, Stinger, the Commander says to Maverick, "Your family name ain't the best in the Navy. You need to be doing it better and cleaner than the other guy" (Tolkan, 1986). So, if this is you, you're not doomed, but you do need to be aware that you will need to follow your regimen more cleanly than the person who hasn't experienced an increase in fat cell number. It's important to come to a place of acceptance about this. As a scientist with over 85,000 hours of laboratory experience, I've witnessed the implications of these physiological realities. So, although you got yourself into this situation, take my hand and let's get you out of it together.

Do you see yourself in Martin's story? Can you relate to his fears and sense of powerlessness to make any meaningful improvements in your health? Please take time to look through Martin's reports and perhaps even listen to him share his story.

160 Solving the Weight Loss Puzzle

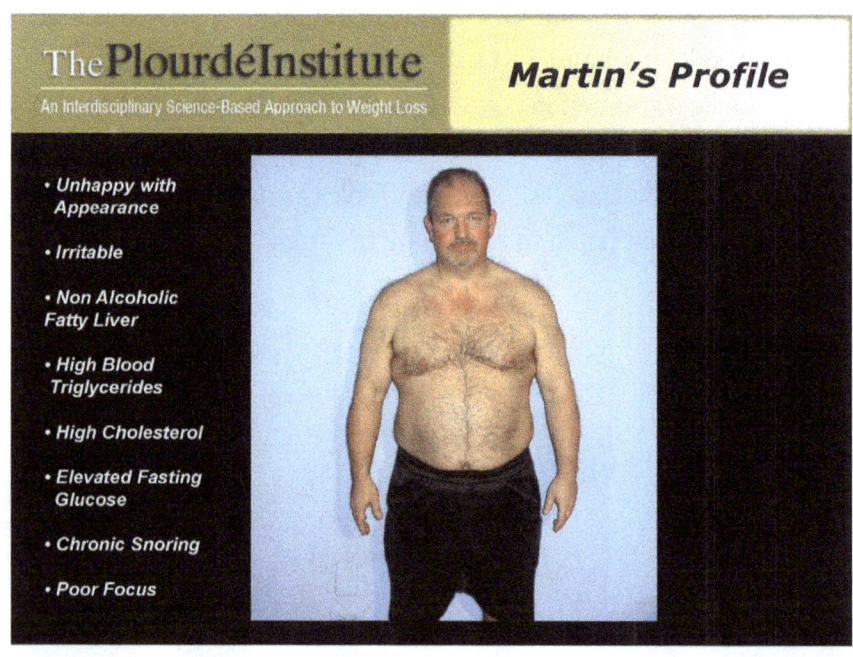

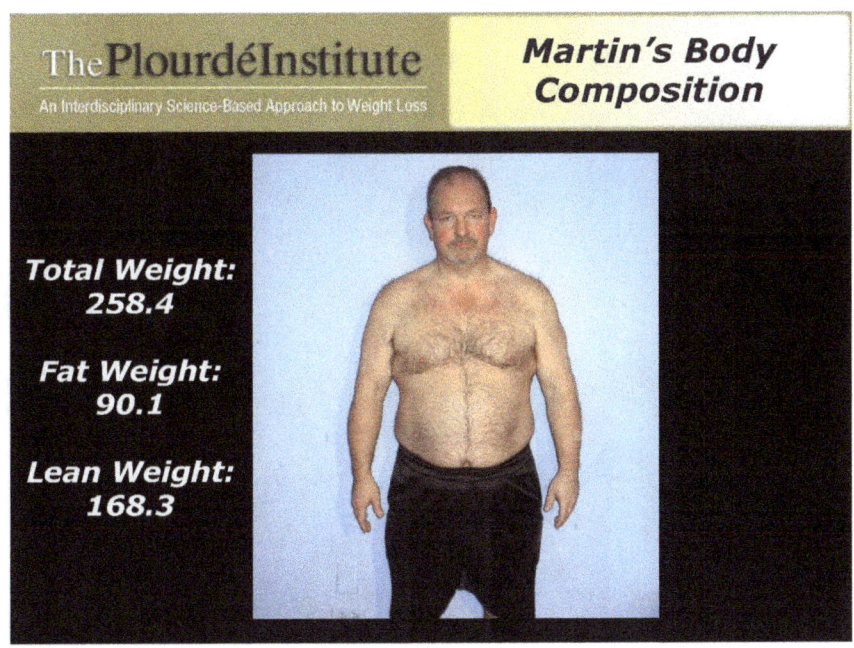

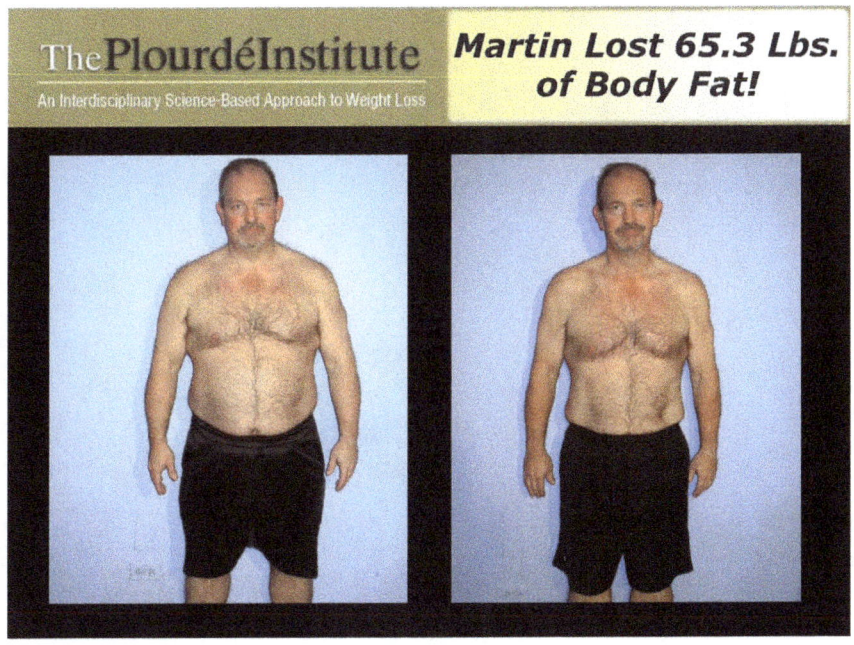

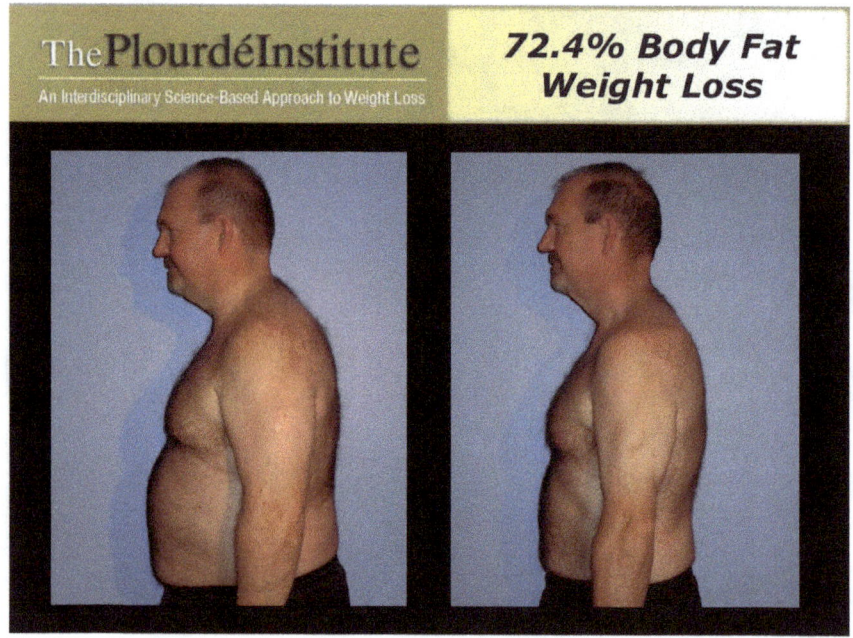

The Plourdé Institute
An Interdisciplinary Science-Based Approach to Weight Loss

Historical Evaluation of Adiposity

Name _____ Martin _____ Date ___ 2/11/2022 ___

Condition of Adiposity	Baseline	Peak	Current	Goal - 50%	Goal - 60%	Goal - 71%	Goal - 75%	Goal - 80%
Body Fat %	18.0	43.5	34.9	26.3	21.9	16.7	14.7	12.1
Fat Weight	36.9	121.9	90.1	61.0	48.8	35.4	30.5	24.4
Lean Weight	168.1	158.1	168.3	171.0	173.7	176.4	176.4	176.4
Total Weight	205.0	280.0	258.4	232.0	222.5	211.8	206.9	200.8
Age	18	49	51	51	51	51	51	51
# of Adipocytes	27.9	46.1	46.1	46.1	46.1	46.1	46.1	46.1

Fat Weight Increase of ___ 85.0 ___ lbs. = ___ 230.4 ___ %

Type of Lipogenesis =

(Type 1) Adipocyte Hypertrophy ☐

(Type 2) Adipocyte Hyperplastic Hypertrophy (Both Types) ☐

Fat Weight Reduction Goal: 29.2 lbs = 32.4 %
41.3 lbs = 45.9 %
54.7 lbs = 60.8 %
59.6 lbs = 66.2 %
65.7 lbs = 72.9 %

Estimated Range of Reduction Phase = __7-10__ months

Copyright © 2023 David Plourdé, Ph.D.

The Plourdé Institute
An Interdisciplinary Science-Based Approach to Weight Loss

BODY COMPOSITION PROGRESS CHART
CLIENT NAME: MARTIN   GOAL FAT WEIGHT: 24.4

DATE	TOTAL WEIGHT	FAT WEIGHT	LEAN WEIGHT	FAT LOSS	% FAT LOSS	TOTAL FAT LOSS
2/11/2020	280.0	121.9	158.1			
2/11/2022	258.4	90.1	168.3	31.76	-26.1%	31.76
3/12/2022	241.2	71.6	169.5	18.48	-20.5%	50.24
4/9/2022	230.3	59.7	170.7	11.95	-16.7%	62.19
5/14/2022	219.1	46.9	172.3	12.80	-21.5%	74.99
6/18/2022	209.8	36.3	173.5	10.59	-22.6%	85.58
7/23/2022	202.6	28.3	174.3	7.99	-22.0%	93.58
9/30/2022	200.2	24.8	175.4	3.45	-12.2%	97.03

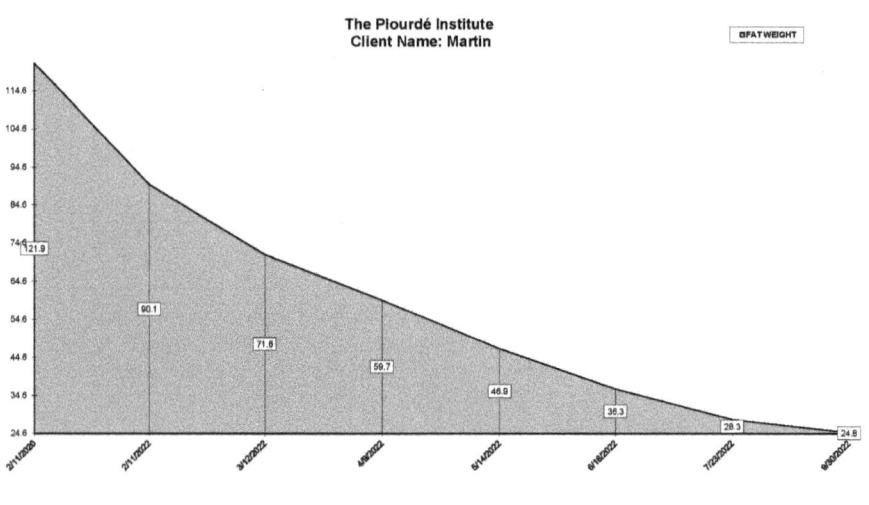

Subsection: Understanding Inflammation

Let me make one other very important point: when someone has a 200, 300, 400 or 500 percent increase in body fat over the course of their adult life, it is essentially impossible for this outcome to occur without continuously elevated insulin (as a hormone, insulin signals hormone-sensitive lipase for fat synthesis in the fat cell).

The problem with this fact is that even slightly elevated insulin over the course of time produces an inflammatory state in the body. This inflammatory state will manifest with stiffness and swelling throughout the body. This is a musculoskeletal symptom. However, the inflammatory conditions don't stop with your knees, hips, fingers, or neck, but extend to peripheral vascular as well as cardiovascular inflammation. This may be an explanation as to why type II diabetics are susceptible to strokes, heart attacks, and diabetic neuropathy.

When the body is in an inflammatory state, the blood vessels at the extremities are the smallest, and therefore are the first to show signs of vascular plaque or the occlusion of blood flow. You can see it in the toes, but people will also notice it with their vision, their hearing, and even blood flow to the genitals. The epidemic of erectile dysfunction among men is a result in part due to decreased blood flow due to plaque accumulation in the smaller blood vessels within the genitals.

Let me reiterate: I am not a medical doctor. I'm a Ph.D. scientist. My wheelhouse is chemistry within the field of nutrition and the understanding of cellular respiration or metabolism within the field of exercise physiology, and I have observed thousands of people over the course of time with very careful monitoring. I operate a laboratory. When people are guided by science regarding precise changes in diet, exercise, stress management, etc., the body can heal itself. I'm not promising that accumulated plaque at the peripheral blood vessels or heart is going to reverse, but what I *can* say is that the inflammatory conditions may slow or entirely cease, impacting the progression of disease dramatically. I know this to be true because many of the thousands of people who have come to see me over the years work closely with their personal physician and have documented these outcomes.

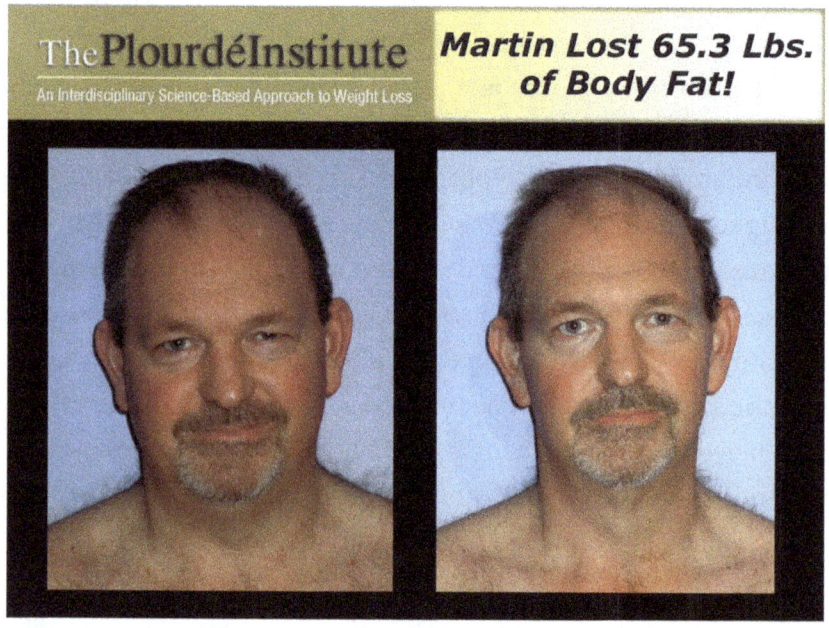

The inflammatory conditions that I'm speaking of are always visible in the face. As people gain fat over the course of their lives and have continuously elevated insulin, inflammatory conditions show up loud and clear. The face will appear swollen and puffy. It's not pleasant. The good news is there's an incredible anti-aging benefit when you dramatically control insulin: inflammatory conditions stop in their tracks. The facial features that you saw in yourself when you were younger begin to emerge, and it's an incredible feeling that many of my clients have enjoyed.

▶▶▶ Let me illustrate another example of a client success story that demonstrates the connection between increasing body fat over the course of adult life and disease progression. I introduce you to Duane. He is a forty-six-year-old African American successful business owner. He founded an outdoor living architectural design firm with his lovely wife, Isabel. He grew this business from nothing to a multimillion-dollar company, and has been living a great life for years. Despite all of his success, he was failing with his health profoundly.

While shopping for an airplane, he met a former client of mine, Tom, who lost significant amounts of body fat in 2011 (see Tom's before and after picture below). Somehow, in that moment, the subject of Duane's health predicament came up. In his effort to get his pilot's license, the Federal Aviation Administration (FAA) denied him because his blood sugar was dangerously high: 350+. Although he sought the guidance of medical doctors and dietitians, his condition got progressively worse. For him, it was the death of his dream to become a pilot.

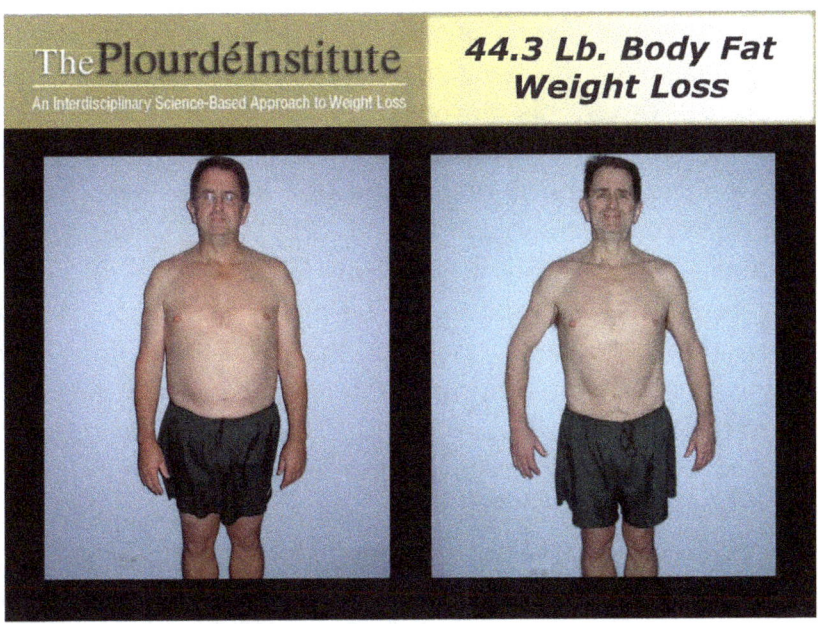

Somehow, he refused to give up on his dream. Spontaneously, Duane uncharacteristically shared vulnerably about his situation. Tom made a bold statement, "There's only one guy you need to talk to right now. It's Dr. Plourdé from The Plourdé Institute. He'll teach you exactly what you need to do to reduce your body fat and correct your blood sugar problems."

He proceeded to share my contact information with him and Duane promptly reached out to me. Without any delay, Duane moved forward with a phone intake, assessing his clinical need for weight loss as well as his psychological and emotional readiness for change. He checked all the boxes, and we scheduled for him to come in for an assessment. Here's what we learned:

At the age of eighteen years old, Duane weighed 165 pounds, with only 13.2 pounds of body fat. Fast forward to the age of thirty-four. Duane weighed 258 pounds, with 111.5 pounds of body fat. This represented a 98.3 pound body fat weight gain, or a 744.7 percent increase in body fat. During the assessment, I observed that a disproportionate amount of his body fat gain was intra-abdominal. His blood tests indicated major signs of non-alcoholic fatty liver. During this period, his blood sugar was above 350. To say this was dangerous was an understatement.

In short order, his body fat reduced to 37.8 pounds, representing a 74-pound fat loss from his peak fat weight. This was a 66 percent body fat weight loss. Duane's blood sugar went from consistently over 350 to 120. When Duane visited his medical doctor, sadly, he was browbeaten. Duane refused to inject insulin and wanted to solve his problems by more natural means. He fundamentally believed that he lacked information. He was seeking someone to mentor him regarding nutrition, chemistry, metabolism, and health. His persistence, tenacity, humility, and receptivity paid enormous dividends. As you look through his reports, you will plainly see that not only is he unrecognizable physically, but more importantly, his blood tests show his liver function, blood sugar, and endocrine physiology (hormone function) normalized. I don't mean to be hyperbolic, but you could say, in many ways, this outcome borders on the miraculous.

The Plourdé Institute
An Interdisciplinary Science-Based Approach to Weight Loss

Historical Evaluation of Adiposity

Name: Duane   Date: 5/11/2022

Condition of Adiposity	Baseline	Peak	Current	Goal - 50%	Goal - 60%	Goal - 71%	Goal - 75%	Goal - 80%
Body Fat %	8.0	43.2	34.7	27.7	23.2	17.7	15.6	12.9
Fat Weight	13.2	111.5	75.7	55.8	44.6	32.3	27.9	22.3
Lean Weight	151.8	146.5	142.5	145.2	147.9	150.6	150.6	150.6
Total Weight	165.0	258.0	218.2	201.0	192.5	182.9	178.5	172.9
Age	18	34	46	46	46	46	46	46
# of Adipocytes	10.0	42.1	42.1	42.1	42.1	42.1	42.1	42.1

Fat Weight Increase of __98.3__ lbs. = __744.7__ %

Type of Lipogenesis =

(Type 1) Adipocyte Hypertrophy ☐

(Type 2) Adipocyte Hyperplastic Hypertrophy (Both Types) ☐

Fat Weight Reduction Goal: 20.0 lbs = 26.4 %
　　　　　　　　　　　　　　 31.1 lbs = 41.1 %
　　　　　　　　　　　　　　 43.4 lbs = 57.3 %
　　　　　　　　　　　　　　 47.8 lbs = 63.2 %
　　　　　　　　　　　　　　 53.4 lbs = 70.5 %

Estimated Range of Reduction Phase = __7-9__ months

Copyright © 2023 David Plourdé, Ph.D.

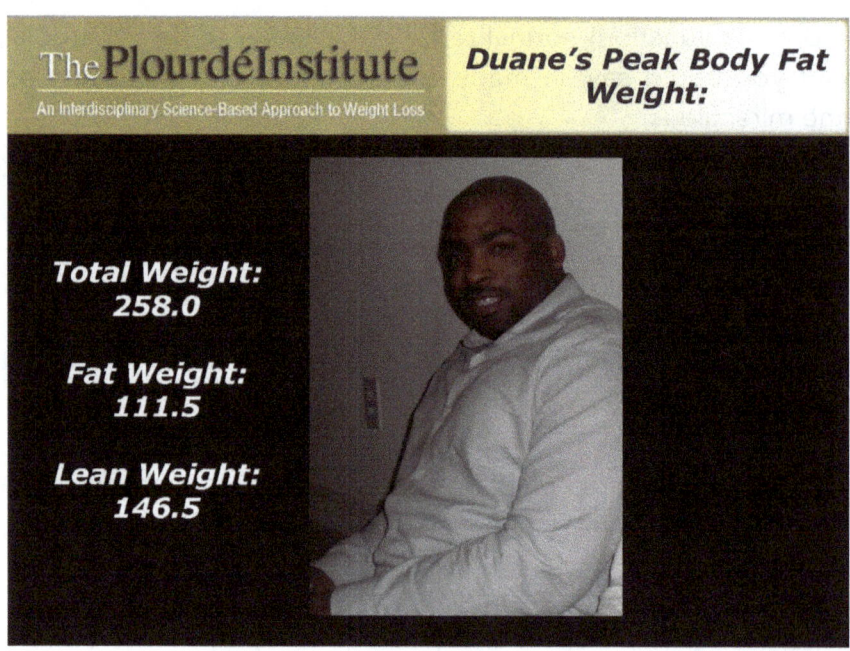

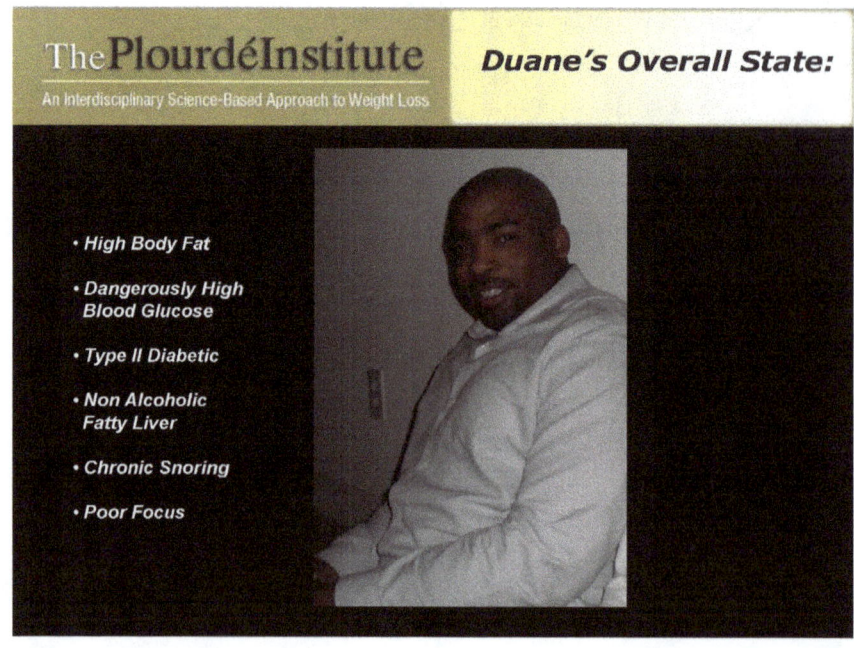

The Plourdé Institute
An Interdisciplinary Science-Based Approach to Weight Loss

BODY COMPOSITION PROGRESS CHART

CLIENT NAME: DUANE **GOAL FAT WEIGHT: 32.3**

DATE	TOTAL WEIGHT	FAT WEIGHT	LEAN WEIGHT	FAT LOSS	% FAT LOSS	TOTAL FAT LOSS
5/11/2010	258.0	111.5	146.5			
5/11/2022	218.2	75.7	142.5	35.79	-32.1%	35.79
6/17/2022	205.4	61.5	143.9	14.19	-18.8%	49.98
9/23/2022	196.8	49.3	147.5	12.18	-19.8%	62.16
3/10/2023	191.7	42.6	149.1	6.71	-13.6%	68.87
8/10/2023	189.5	37.8	151.7	4.77	-11.2%	73.65

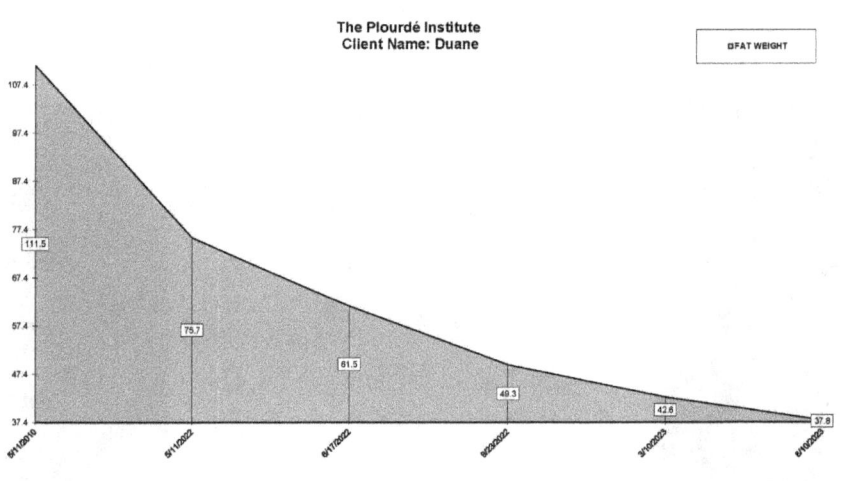

172   Solving the Weight Loss Puzzle

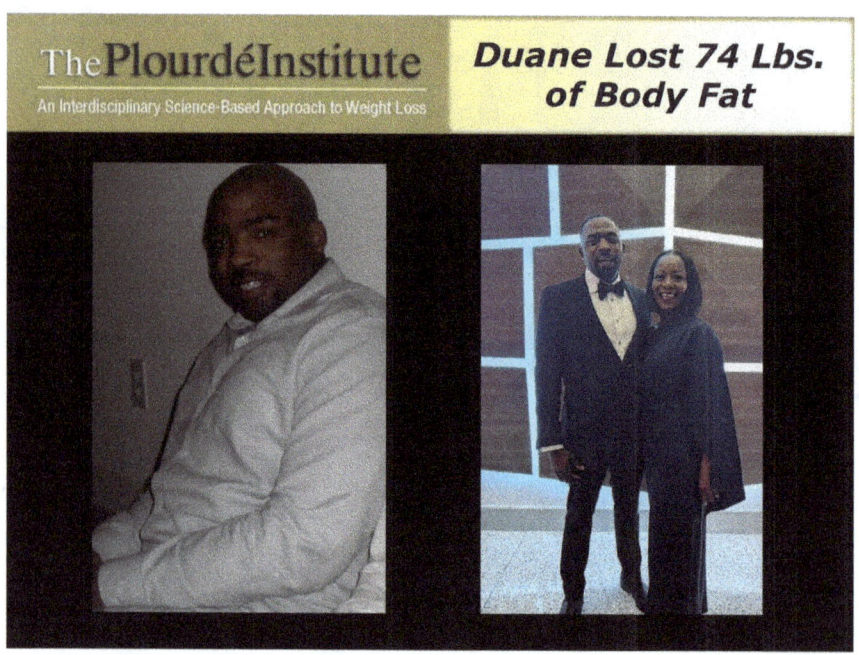

Source: Duane's personal photos shared with permission

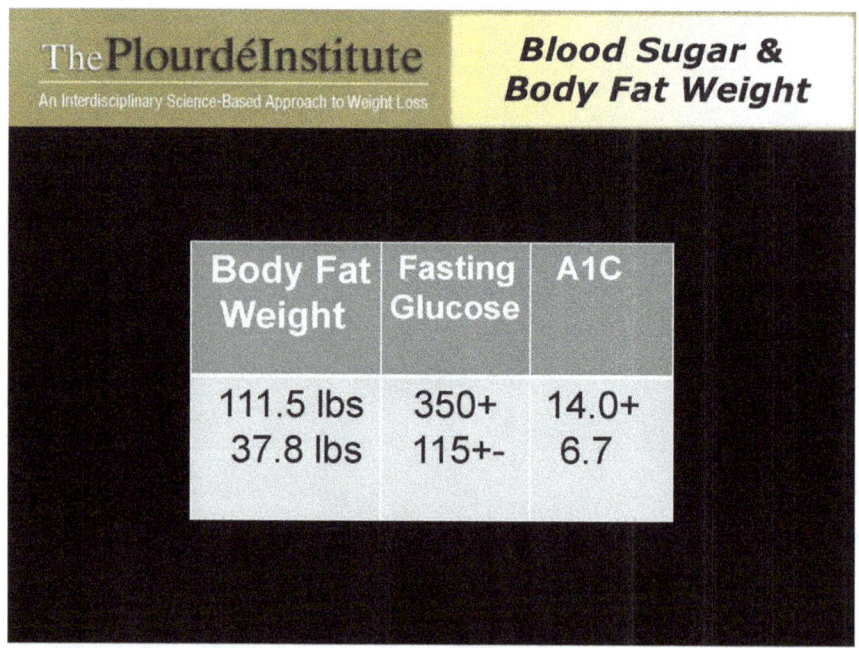

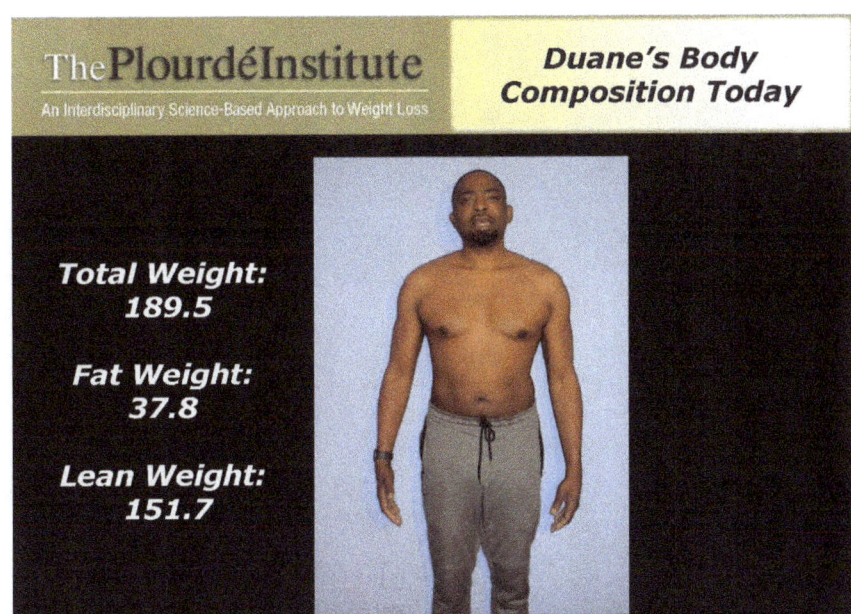

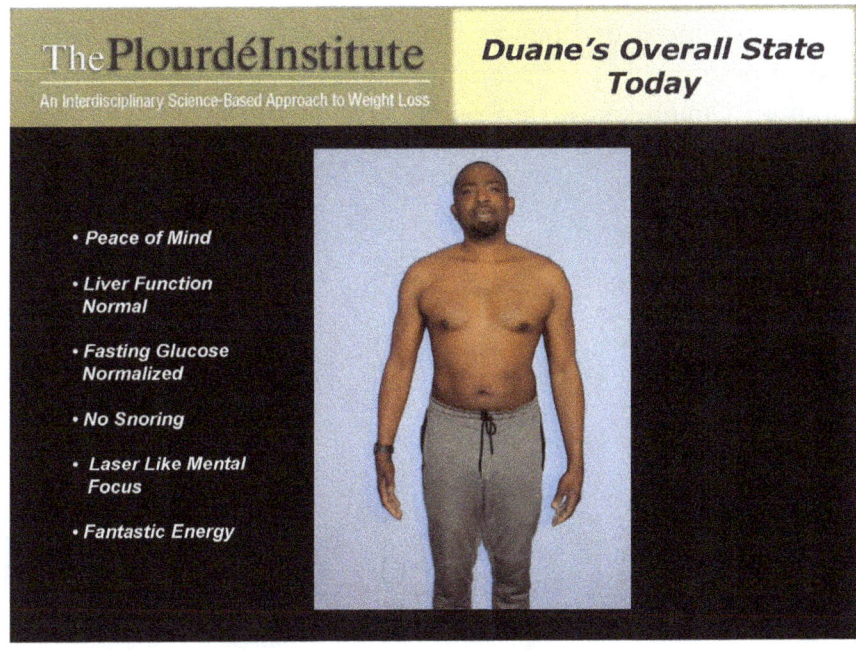

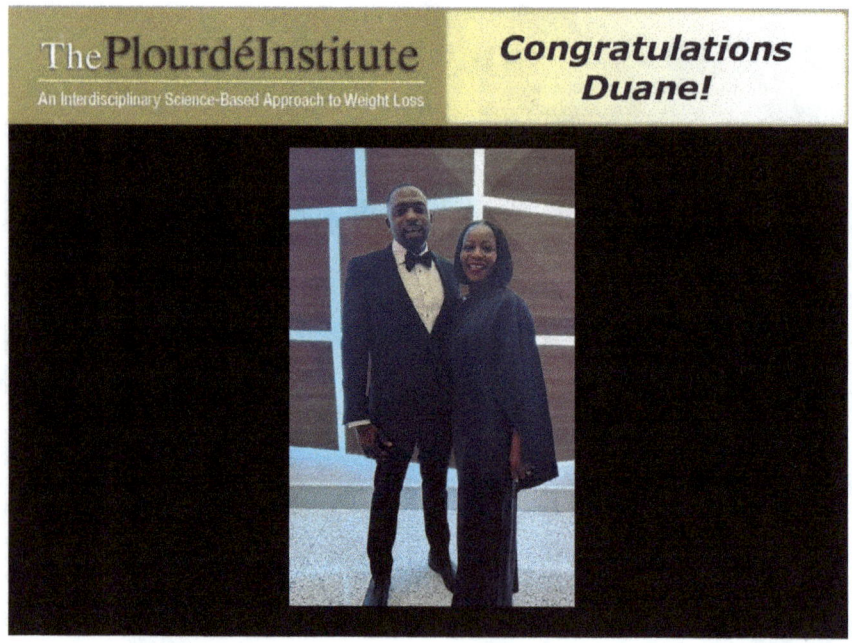

Source: Duane's personal photos shared with permission

One element of Duane's highlight reel is that after having experienced this profound health transformation, the FAA granted Duane his private pilot's license and made his dream a reality! ▶▶▶

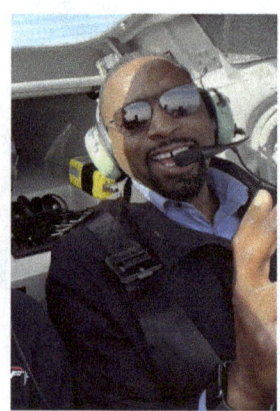

Source: Duane's personal photo shared with permission

When the private clients of The Plourdé Institute meet our compliance criteria, men lose 71 percent to 80 percent of their body fat with a 95 percent probability. Women lose 61 percent to 73 percent of their peak body fat weight with a 95 percent probability. Many of the comorbidities or diseases associated with high body fat improve. This has been an observable fact that I have monitored for over thirty-three years.

I would like to include a gentle reminder that the version of intellectual property that is being shared in this book may likely result in greater than a 50 percent body fat weight loss. The full breadth of the METHOD and comprehensive trade secrets are disclosed fully only to our private clients. Having said that, you will still greatly benefit from all of the things discussed related to body fat and disease progression.

If no one in your health care network has ever spoken to you this way, I'm not surprised. At Plourdé, we speak a different language. Our goal is to help you understand the science of how your body works. It's been said many times that an idea you don't understand is an idea that's powerless. We go to great lengths to make sure that our clients internalize these concepts, and as a result, feel incredible hope and motivation to actually follow through.

CHAPTER 13

When Food is Your Drug

Over the course of my career, thousands of people have sought my professional guidance. Regardless of who I deal with, the journey always begins with a phone intake to assess the person's clinical need for weight loss, as well as their psychological and emotional readiness for change.

As we delve into the process, we camp out on the subject of their pain. Here are some of the common denominators that people feel: despair or a sense of hopelessness, confusion, frustration, shame, self-loathing, weakness. I could go on, but I think you get the picture. The point that I want to make here is that my clients have expressed deep psychological and emotional agony in their plight; it's a dark place. Can you relate?

The following is a very bold statement, but I have found it to be true. If you only throw physical science at the problem of unsuccessful weight loss, but fail to address your interior life, you might as well never even begin.

I think it's fair to say that in most cases, the biggest obstacle in our weight loss journey is ourselves, and a big part of the solution is to get out of your own way. Do you ever find yourself eating at night when you're not hungry, or eating well past full, or binging? If you're anything like my clients, you've probably asked yourself the following question a thousand times, "Why do I keep doing these things?"

Is it possible that food is a drug for you? That's the case for many of my clients.

Let's begin this chapter by both sharing my definition of addiction and unpacking the physiology of addiction. First, the definition.

Definition of Addiction

Addiction is a state of dependence on something or someone in order to feel normalcy, pleasure, or relief, even in spite of colossal negative consequences, usually with an inability to stop engaging or using the substance or external stimulant. It's also associated with deep psychological and emotional incongruence, where a person desires to stop using but can't stop and often feels a multitude of negative emotions: anger, frustration, confusion, and shame because of his or her inability to control their impulses.

Second, a brief explanation of the physiology of addiction.

The Physiology of Addiction

The need for something external to produce a change in one's psychological, emotional, and overall physical state: the act of using evokes neurological and endocrine responses—the release of dopamine and serotonin in the brain and the release of epinephrine and norepinephrine from the adrenal glands, with the intended outcome of inducing a state of pleasure and or relief physiologically. The pleasure one receives from using can make abstinence very difficult, and in the mind of the user it may seem impossible to stop.

My First Observations of Addiction

My first observations of addiction occurred in 1994. This is where the story begins:

▶▶▶ Melinda arrived at The Plourdé Institute on Tuesday, June 8, 1993, for her weight loss assessment. At that time, we evaluated her clinical need for weight loss, as well as her psychological and emotional readiness for change. At the end of the assessment, we both agreed the program was a good fit for her, and that she was ready to commit to changing her life. Through the course of her journey, she lost nearly eighty-five pounds of body fat.

In late June of 1994, Melinda walked into my office and sat down for her weekly session. She went on to ask me for a very personal favor. She openly confessed that she thought she was an alcoholic. She asked me if I would hold her accountable for going to AA meetings. I told her of course I would. The following week she showed up for her appointment with me. Her hair was disheveled, she smelled like smoke and she looked like she had been up all night. I simply asked her, "How are those meetings going?"

She said, "Well, I haven't been to any."

Uncharacteristically, I replied, "Today is your last session. You asked me to hold you accountable. You either go to meetings or we're done here."

Melinda was stunned by my sternness, but I believed, intuitively, that she needed tough love. She agreed. This interaction occurred right before the July 4th weekend of 1994.

The following week she came in for her weekly session and sat down in the chair in my office and immediately began to sob uncontrollably. I asked her, "What's wrong?!"

She answered in between sobs, "Remember that intervention we had last week?"

I said, "Of course I do."

She went on to say, "I was at work over the weekend (Melinda was a server in a very successful microbrewery, of all places) and on Saturday night, one of my coworkers, Jodie, asked me to go out and party after work. I quickly said, 'Sure, I'll go out, but I'm not going to drink.' As I walked away from Jodie, I thought to myself, 'My sobriety is in such a fragile state. I probably need to say no.' So later that evening, I went up to Jodie and said, 'On second thought, I'm feeling tired and I think I'm just going to go home and go to bed early tonight. I'm sorry.'"

She went on to explain, "When I came back to work after the July 4th weekend, one of my other coworkers quickly came up to me and said, 'Did you hear what happened to Jodie?!' I said, 'No! What happened?"

The coworker said Jodie was involved in a head-on car collision. Melinda and I realized that, had she gone out and partied that night with Jodie, she would've likely been sitting in the passenger seat and may have been killed. When I heard this from Melinda, I was shocked. I realized that the intervention we had had the previous week may have very well saved her life. ▶▶▶

That moment will be forever imprinted in the depths of my being. At that instant, I realized the magnitude of potential destructiveness that addiction yields. I have never been the same since. I've made it a point to teach the "Twelve Steps" of Alcoholics Anonymous® (www.aa.org 1952, 1953, 1981) when appropriate in my program for the purpose of food addiction recovery.

I've also had the privilege of working with many successful men and women who faithfully embrace the "Twelve Steps" in their own sobriety path. These people have inspired me throughout my career, demonstrating uncommon humility, courage, and faith. Their lives are a testimony to the incontrovertible truths at the core of the Steps.

Now, let's talk about you. Perhaps you've been struggling with a weight problem most of your life. You may have tried different programs and different diets. You've seen a therapist and worked with a trainer. You may have tried a semaglutide and stopped because you had side effects. You're not getting traction. To say that you're frustrated is a huge understatement. You keep trying but you can't seem to change your behavior. You want to but you can't. You try, and you try, and you try, but you're not making any progress.

You may still be wondering: what *really* makes THE PLOURDE METHOD℠ different from other weight loss programs? One major difference is that we look at the weight loss journey through the lens of a sobriety path. In this section of the book, I will share a fresh perspective on the most successful sobriety plan ever created—the "Twelve Steps" of AA. Here, we apply the Steps in the context of food addiction.

The following is a brief overview of Steps one through three and how they relate to food addiction recovery:

Step One
"We admitted that we were powerless over *our dependencies*—that our lives had become unmanageable."

You've hit bottom. In other words, you have a problem and you know you can't fix it. You've come to the end of your capacity. You've tried everything in your power to succeed in this area, but nothing is working. If you look at your life like a pie chart, you might have a beautiful pie chart. Many of the slivers of the pie of your life are in a nice, neat order . . . except one. This one department of your life is in complete disarray. It keeps you up at night. It preoccupies you continuously.

Here are a few signs that you might have an addictive relationship with food:

> *You consistently eat at night when you're not hungry.*
>
> *You consistently eat well past full.*
>
> *You binge regularly or at least occasionally.*
>
> *You don't like the way you look.*
>
> *You don't like the way you feel.*

You don't like the way you feel about yourself.

You avoid intimacy.

You can't stand your picture being taken.

You're confused.

You're frustrated.

You're mad at yourself and ask, "How did I let myself get to this place?"

You feel fearful about the trajectory of your health.

You're approaching or already have type II diabetes.

Your blood pressure is elevated.

You snore and may suffer from obstructive sleep apnea.

You may have difficulty breathing.

You're stiff and sore and your body is showing signs of arthritis.

When you think about the trajectory of your health in another ten years you're wondering, "Am I even going to be here?"

You're overweight and feel that this area of your life is out of control.

If you agree with several of these statements, you may struggle with food addiction.

Step Two:
"Came to believe that a Power greater than ourselves could restore us to sanity."

Perhaps, the one thing you haven't done yet is ask God sincerely for His help to restore you to sanity, but you may now be realizing it's time to do that. But how? In the Bible, Jesus explained it in the

Gospel of Matthew: "Ask and it will be given to you; seek and you will find; knock and the door will be opened to you." (Matthew 7:7 NIV)

Perhaps you could consider praying: "Please help me, God, to restore my life to sanity. Please give me self-control, peace, joy, and self-respect."

The essence of Step Two is that although you don't have the power to solve your problem, God does. I'd like to illustrate the power of Step Two by recounting in my own words the story of Gideon from chapters six and seven of the book of Judges in the Old Testament of the Bible.

▶▶▶ In chapter six, it begins with the following phrase: "Again, Israel did evil in the eyes of the Lord . . ." (Judges 6:1 NIV).

In his anger, God had allowed a powerful army made up of the Midianites, the Amalekites, and other eastern peoples to oppress the people of Israel. This was an army of over 125,000 heavily armed, fully trained men with an immense cavalry. This military force robbed Israel of all of its produce, livestock, and possessions. The people were so impoverished that they sought refuge in mountain caves to escape the brutality of their oppressors.

The angel of the Lord, which many believe was the pre-incarnate Jesus Himself, appeared to a humble man named Gideon. At this moment, Gideon was making an effort to hide wheat from the opposing forces in a winepress. Sitting in a pool of self-pity, doubt, and fear, the angel of the Lord said to Gideon, "The LORD is with you, mighty warrior."

Gideon feebly responded, "Wait a minute, don't you know who you're talking to? I come from the weakest clan of Israel. I have nothing and I am nothing."

The angel of the Lord went on to encourage Gideon, making it clear to him that he was God's chosen deliverer to defeat this massive army.

Faced with colossal doubt, Gideon sought God's reassurance

by asking for a miracle—it was actually the same miracle twice. He would place a fleece in the winepress and ask that in the morning the floor of the winepress be dry, but the fleece be wet with dew. And the next day, the Lord did so. In weakness, Gideon sought assurance again, "Please don't be angry with me, but I'd like one more test with the fleece. Tomorrow morning, please let the fleece be dry, but the floor of the winepress be wet with dew." And the Lord did so.

Because Gideon was overwhelmed with self-doubt, the angel of the Lord said to Gideon, "Go in the strength you have." (Note that he didn't say go in the strength *you don't have*.) Then the Spirit of the Lord came upon Gideon, and he blew the shofar (an ancient musical instrument made from the horn of a ram), calling all men of military age to fight against the opposing military forces, and 32,000 fighting men showed up at Gideon's doorstep.

Strangely, the Lord said to Gideon, "You have too many men for me to bless you. In order that Israel may not boast that in her own strength she defeated this army, make an announcement, 'If any one of you are overwhelmed with fear, you can go home.'"

At that time, 22,000 men embarrassingly admitted they were scared and proceeded to go home.

Surprisingly, the Lord said to Gideon, "You *still* have too many men for me to bless you," and went on to explain who would stay to fight and who would go home. The Lord directed 9,700 men to go home, and with only 300 men, He promised the complete annihilation of the Midianites, the Amalekites, and the other eastern peoples.

It's important to point out that although Gideon knew he was talking with God face-to-face, he was *still* overwhelmed with insecurity, fear, and massive self-doubt. In an effort to reassure Gideon, the Lord instructed him to go down to the opposing forces during the change of the guard in the middle of the night. He said to Gideon, "I'm going to let you overhear a conversation that will give you all the reassurance that you need."

Gideon obeyed the Lord and went down to the camp with one of his top lieutenants. As he approached, he overheard a conversation between two of the soldiers. One of them said to the other, "Last night I had a dream. In the dream, a massive barley loaf came rolling down the mountain and completely destroyed the tents of our army."

The other soldier said to him, "This can only mean one thing: God has turned us over to the hand of Gideon and we are doomed." When Gideon heard these words, he was filled with hope, faith, and confidence.

Shortly after this, *with just 300 men*, the Lord instructed him to surround the enemy's camp. Each of Gideon's men would be holding a torch covered by a clay pot, and at Gideon's signal, the men of Israel would smash the clay pots, raise their torch, and say the following words, "A sword for the Lord and for Gideon!"

At their utterance, the army of over 125,000 heavily armed and military-trained men, in complete confusion, attacked *each other* and the entire enemy army was decimated without Gideon's men lifting a finger. ▶▶▶

Can you see yourself in this story? Are you facing an insurmountable challenge, feeling entirely incapable of succeeding? Well, you're in good company. Could it be that God has allowed this problem (let me be clear: He did not *cause* the problem) to help you come to your senses?

That's what the Apostle Paul suggests in his letter to the church of Rome in chapter seven and eight of Romans in the Bible. In chapter seven, Paul expresses vulnerably an undisclosed pattern of behavior that he could not seem to stop. You can read the chapter and hear the depth of his struggle and his humble confession that he was completely incapable of ceasing an unproductive behavior.

The Apostle Paul suggests that there may be a divine purpose in your pain in Romans 8:20. It is paraphrased here: the creation (humanity) was subjected to these types of frustrations, not by their own choice, but God allowed it in the hope that they would be liberated from their bondage to decay and be brought into the glorious freedom of the children of God.

You see, God has all the power you need to help you find freedom, better health, joy, and self-respect. In many of Paul's letters, also called the Epistles, Paul systematically explains that a right-standing with God comes *not* from human effort, human works, or human righteousness, but rather it comes by faith in the Savior of the world, Jesus Christ. I'm not inferring that eating unhealthy food or being overweight is sinful or immoral, because Jesus very clearly states that it is not what goes into our mouths that makes us sinful, but rather what comes from our hearts. He goes on to list a series of immoralities. Food is not moral. However, for some people the lifelong patterns of incongruent behavior and the consequences of those behaviors on our mental, emotional, and physical health are glaring and painful realities.

Is it possible that the freedom you are seeking, that you have sought with all your might but have failed to obtain, will come to you not by trying harder but rather by faith? That's precisely what I am saying. Let's revisit the wording of Step Two one more time before we move on to Step Three: "Came to believe that a Power greater than ourselves could restore us to sanity."

Step Three:
"Made a decision to turn our will and our lives over to the care of God . . ."

The Bible, in the book of Genesis, states that we were created in the image of God. What does that mean? It means that we're like God. God created us with the power of free will.

The word "will" is defined in the 1913 version of *Webster's Dictionary* as:

> *The power of choosing; the faculty or endowment of the soul by which it is capable of choosing; the faculty or power of the mind by which we decide to do or not to do; the power or faculty of preferring or selecting one of two or more objects.*

Simply stated, it's the power to choose. However, from the beginning of creation, we see the human "chooser" malfunctioning.

▶▶▶ In my own recounting of a portion of Genesis 2 from the Bible, God tells Adam, "I created all of this for you. You can have everything. I did it just for you. However, you may not eat from the tree in the middle of the garden, the tree of the knowledge of good and evil. If you eat of it, you will surely die."

Satan enters the picture as a beautiful creature seducing Adam's wife, Eve, with the physical beauty of the apple, its luscious taste, and the promise to be like God. He tempted her on every level. In First John chapter 2, verse 16, John describes that there are three categories of sin: "lust of the flesh, lust of the eyes, and the pride of life—comes not from the Father from the world." (NIV) We see that Eve was tested in all three areas.

Adam stands at her side passively, in weakness, and allows this seduction and deception to occur. He sheepishly joins in and takes a bite of the apple. At that point, everything unravels.

We see the first family spiral out of control. God delivers consequences to Adam and Eve when he says, "Your desire will be for your husband and he will rule over you." (Genesis 3:16, NIV).

This may be interpreted that there will be a continuous battle for dominance in male and female intimate relationships. God also says to Eve, "You will suffer great pain in childbearing." (Genesis 3:16, NIV).

To Adam he said, "Because you listened to your wife and ate from the tree about which I commanded you, 'You must not eat of it,' "Cursed is the ground because of you; through painful toil you will eat of it all the days of your life." (Genesis 3:17, NIV) This may be interpreted that men would struggle in their efforts to provide for their families.

Because of these circumstances, death became part of the reality of human existence, and they were subsequently kicked out of the Garden of Eden—never to be allowed to return. This death was not just a physical death, but perhaps even more importantly, a spiritual death, which meant that people would live in the absence of God's presence.

This reality was manifested with the further unraveling of human relationships in the first family when Cain kills his brother Abel when overcome by feelings of jealousy and anger. And from that point it just continues to get worse. Fast forward to today. We see the human choosing mechanism (or will) is totally malfunctioning. People often make choices that make absolutely no sense. We see our society crumbling before our eyes and we don't know why.

Let me begin by apologizing for some redundancy, as it's highly relevant to explaining the mystery of Step Three. I'd like to look at some of the Apostle Paul's words, which he wrote so eloquently in his letter to the church in Rome in Romans chapter 7, starting with verse 15:

> *I do not understand what I do. For what I want to do I do not do, but what I hate I do. And if I do what I do not want to do, I agree that the law is good. As it is, it is no longer I myself who do it, but it is sin living in me. For I know that good itself does not dwell in me, that is, in my sinful nature. For I have the desire to do what is good, but I cannot carry it out. For I do not do the good I want to do, but the evil I do not want to*

> *do—this I keep on doing. Now if I do what I do not want to do, it is no longer I who do it, but it is sin living in me that does it. So I find this law at work: Although I want to do good, evil is right there with me. For in my inner being I delight in God's law; but I see another law at work in me, waging war against the law of my mind and making me a prisoner of the law of sin at work within me. What a wretched man I am! Who will rescue me from this body that is subject to death? Thanks be to God, who delivers me through Jesus Christ our Lord!* (Romans 7:15-25 NIV)

If you can relate to Paul's internal dialogue—and I'll bet you can—then keep reading. Maybe your self-talk sounds like this, "Ugh, I shouldn't have done that. I need to stop. I'm going to start tomorrow," but you keep playing this mental mind game every day—day after day. It's like you have two natures (or two minds) inside of you: a higher mind that is rational and sane and a lower mind that is irrational and totally counterproductive.

We have already defined, in essence, the power to choose. So, when we take a closer look at Step Three, "Made a decision . . ." the root word of decision is "cision" which means cut. The prefix "de-" means away from. So, "decision" can also be thought of as cutting off from all other options in a specific course of action. In other words, when we make a *real* decision, we are burning the ships. We are literally eliminating all other options and boldly moving in a specific and new direction. Let's continue.

"Made a decision to turn our will and our lives over . . ." We realize that our "chooser" has been fundamentally malfunctioning for perhaps our entire lives. We are literally incapable of straightening our own paths. As we face the pain and the multitude of consequences that may include deep psychological and emotional pain, along with physical ailments related to our health and our lifestyle, we have the opportunity to come to our senses and make a choice to surrender our "chooser."

If you feel similarly to what I just described, this could be a suggested prayer for you: "Lord, I am entirely incapable of straightening my path, and the only way my life path will ever get straight is if You come in and straighten it for me. I'm asking You now, through the power of your Spirit, to help me make better decisions."

In Orthodox Christianity there is a sacrament we call baptism. It is a public proclamation that "my life as I know it is over. As I go under the water, I put to death my fleshly nature, and as I come out of the water my new life, I live by faith in the Son of God who loved me and delivered Himself up for me."

In application to our sobriety path, this means that we need to get out of our own way and humbly and willfully surrender our lives to Him. But you may say to me, "I've already done that and it didn't work."

Perhaps, for you, more pain will be required before you are truly ready to sincerely and completely work Step Three. My hope is that this is a defining moment for you, so I'm asking you to take my hand in faith and walk with me on this incredible path.

Before we go any further, let me recount Step Three: "Made a decision to turn our will and our lives over to the care of God . . ."

A Note about Food and Morality:

Let me be clear: I'm not saying that eating sugar or junk food is immoral, because it's not. The wisest teacher that ever lived, Jesus Christ, said in Matthew

> *Jesus called the crowd to him and said, "Listen and understand. What goes into someone's mouth does not defile them, but what comes out of their mouth, that is what defiles them . . . .*
>
> *Don't you see that whatever enters the mouth goes into the stomach and then out of the body? But the things that come out of a person's mouth come from the heart, and these defile them. For out of the heart come evil thoughts—murder, adultery, sexual immorality, theft, false testimony, slander."* (Matthew 15:10-11, 17-19 NIV)

So, Jesus makes it very clear that food is not moral and we need to be careful not to be legalistic in our weight loss efforts. As the author of this METHOD, I truly enjoy applying these principles in my own everyday life. Am I absolutely perfect in my execution of them? No. At the same time, I am very committed to applying them most of the time. We will all have moments where we slip and eat things that we really don't want to eat (or that we really DO want to eat, but might not be the best choice for our health). It's important that we not beat ourselves up, but rather give ourselves grace and get back on track.

On the next page you will find the full list of the "Twelve Steps."

Service Material from the General Service Office

THE TWELVE STEPS OF ALCOHOLICS ANONYMOUS®

1. We admitted we were powerless over alcohol—that our lives had become unmanageable.
2. Came to believe that a Power greater than ourselves could restore us to sanity.
3. Made a decision to turn our will and our lives over to the care of God as we understood Him.
4. Made a searching and fearless moral inventory of ourselves.
5. Admitted to God, to ourselves, and to another human being the exact nature of our wrongs.
6. We're entirely ready to have God remove all these defects of character.
7. Humbly asked Him to remove our shortcomings.
8. Made a list of all persons we had harmed, and became willing to make amends to them all.
9. Made direct amends to such people wherever possible, except when to do so would injure them or others.
10. Continued to take personal inventory and when we were wrong promptly admitted it.
11. Sought through prayer and meditation to improve our conscious contact with God as we understood Him, praying only for knowledge of His will for us and the power to carry that out.

12. Having had a spiritual awakening as the result of these steps, we tried to carry this message to alcoholics, and to practice these principles in all our affairs.

Copyright 1952, 1953, 1981 by Alcoholics Anonymous Publishing (now known as Alcoholics Anonymous World Services, Inc.) All rights reserved. The Twelve Steps are explained in the book Alcoholics Anonymous. www.aa.org Rev. 11/21 SM F-121

Source: (www.aa.org, 1952, 1953, 1981)

As you look at the totality of the "Twelve Steps" and their application for food addiction, we can say with certainty that Steps One through Three, as well as steps Eleven and Twelve, clearly apply. However, it could be argued that Steps Four through Ten may not apply. As we contemplate Steps Four through Ten, I think the big idea is this: if there are underlying patterns of immoral incongruence in your life resulting in feelings of shame, fear, guilt, insecurity, self-doubt, etc., it's crucial that you identify these incongruencies and change them. This is because shame and the aforementioned painful emotions can be triggers to self-medicate: efforts to numb ourselves from the gnawing and unrelenting consequences of poor and unproductive choices in our lives. In AA, it is protocol for a person to go through these Steps with a sponsor who has lived by them and demonstrated that the ideas have been internalized and faithfully applied. Likewise, as previously mentioned in the accountability chapter, in the weight loss journey, it's important to have a coach that you can confide in to help you connect the dots of unproductive thought patterns, emotions, and behaviors that have perpetually set you back.

Another gem that I borrow from the sobriety vernacular is the acronym HALT:

Hungry

Angry

Lonely

Tired

The idea here is that when you're red-lining, be it psychologically, emotionally, physically, or in some other way, it's not a question of *if* we are going to go off program, but rather *when* and *how far*. **The principle that is being conveyed here is the importance of avoiding extremes: extreme hunger, extreme sleep deprivation, or any other form of extremeness for that matter.**

In application, I have some ideas on how to maintain what I call your "equilibrium"—a state of peace, joy, and gratitude. In this state, you'll find that you don't need to numb yourself. Why would you? You feel so good, with deep feelings of freedom, joy, and self-respect. It's the definition of feeling congruent. Here are some suggested tools that you can place in your proverbial toolkit:

- ☐ Begin your day with solitude and prayer/meditation.
- ☐ Eat every two and a half hours whether hungry or not.
- ☐ Always forgive. The only person unforgiveness hurts is ourself.
- ☐ Incorporate gentle exercise daily.
- ☐ Seek to connect with others on a meaningful level.
- ☐ Be proactive in your life. Plan ahead to avoid unnecessary crises.
- ☐ Make it a habit to go to bed early.

Another important concept is the subject of emotional intelligence. Emotional intelligence is defined as your ability to precisely identify your feelings at any given moment. For many men and for some women, they lack in this area. In practical terms, this simply means that a person has a limited vocabulary of "feeling words." For example, if I ask a man, "How are you feeling?" He might say, "I feel like crap," but what he really meant was that his feelings were hurt or that he felt disrespected; or maybe he felt threatened, insulted, or humiliated.

My point is that when a person has a limited vocabulary of "feeling words," they will likely be unable to differentiate these painful feelings, resulting in a state of overall numbness. This is a trigger and often leads to patterns of self-medicating ourselves to oblivion. One of my coaches taught me the important principle of "taking out the trash," both psychologically and emotionally, once or twice per week. We all know what happens when we don't take out the trash, right? IT STINKS!

Below, you will find a tool that I share with our clients at The Plourdé Institute called "The Emotional Wheel." It's a resource to help you identify your feelings as you seek to "take out the trash." An exercise that I present to my clients is that as you "take out the trash," make a list of your painful emotions while sitting in a state of solitude. When you've recognized all of the emotions that you are feeling, the next step is to convert this list of painful feelings into a prayer and ask for your "daily bread," which is an element of the Lord's Prayer that Jesus taught and is quoted in the Gospels of Matthew and Luke in the Bible. It essentially means your daily sustenance—physical, psychological, emotional, financial, relational, spiritual, etc. In other words, if your painful emotion is fear, your "daily bread" may be to ask God to help you to trust in Him. If your painful emotion is anger, your "daily bread" may be to ask for the power to forgive. If the painful emotion is insecurity, your "daily bread" might be to ask for inner calmness and confidence. I'll close this section of the book by simply saying this, any time I have sincerely asked God for my "daily bread," He has ALWAYS provided.

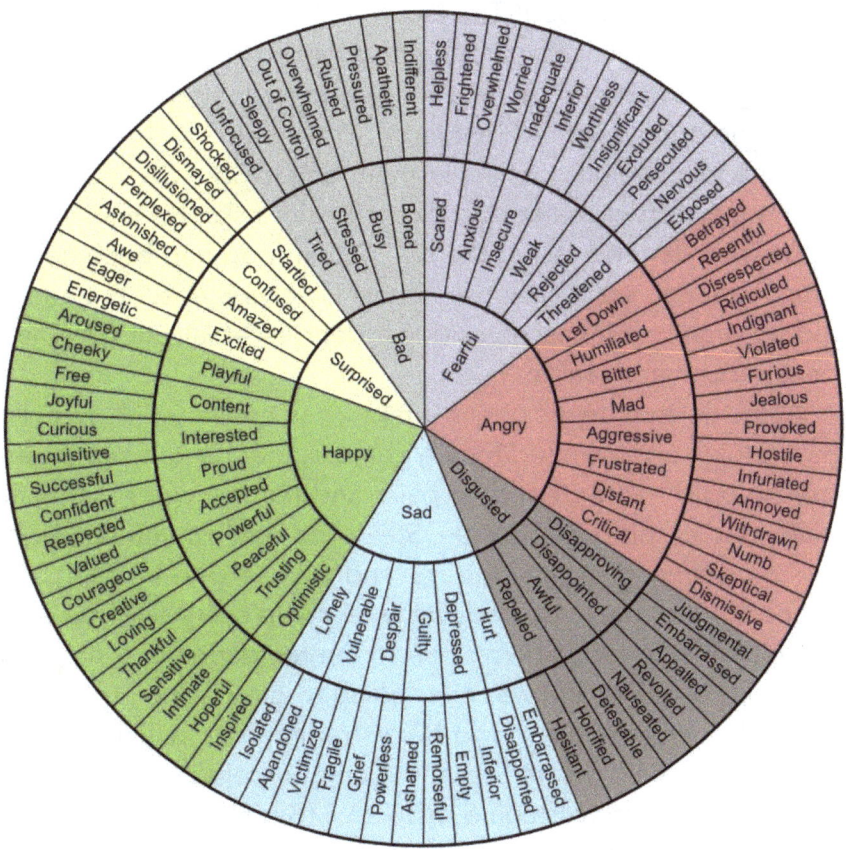

▶▶▶ To help you connect with the idea of food addiction recovery in your own weight loss journey, let me introduce you to Steve. He was forty-six years old, six feet one inch tall, and weighed 380 pounds. This was the most Steve had ever weighed in his life. Although Steve was succeeding in business, happily married to his wife, and had two beautiful daughters, he was in immense pain.

You see, Steve had been overweight for most of his adult life. It had been an issue that had provoked thoughts and feelings of insecurity, self-doubt, shame, and embarrassment—not to mention fear. Steve knew instinctively that he had higher health risks and would ask himself the question, "Do I even have enough life insurance?"

He had learned about The Plourdé Method through his close friend and confidant Martin, who had lost 70 percent of his body fat weight in four months. You may remember his story from earlier in the book. Inspired by Martin, Steve came to The Plourdé Institute for a weight loss assessment on October 22, 2022.

The lab tests revealed significant health risks. He was failing with his health and facing the reality that food had become his drug. In effect, that's step one of the "Twelve Steps." We admitted we were powerless over dependencies—that our lives had become unmanageable.

At the time of Steve's phone intake, I had confirmed that he did have a high clinical need for weight loss, that he had significant psychological and emotional pain, and that he was essentially ready to turn this over. You see, Steve had tried countless weight loss programs, diets, diet books, and worked with trainers, and yet continued to see his body fat level go up every single year of his adult life. In fact, Steve came to the realization that the only way this part of his life was ever going to get back on track was if a higher power came in to help straighten it for him. That is Step Two of the "Twelve Steps": "Came to believe that a power greater than ourselves could restore us to sanity."

Throughout the course of Steve's weight loss assessment, I carefully and methodically explained our scientific method but also addressed the fact that we would have to do some serious work on his interior life, addressing not only the psychology of eating behavior but also the addictive nature of his relationship with food.

That's where Step Three came in: "Made a decision to turn our will and our lives over to the care of God . . ." As previously outlined in this chapter, I needed to hear from Steve that he was ready to get out of his own way.

You might remember the movie *Jerry Maguire* (Crowe, 1996). There's a scene in the movie where Rod Tidwell, an undersized, underrated star wide receiver for the Arizona Cardinals was having a heartfelt conversation with his agent, Jerry Maguire. You see, Rod realized that his wheelhouse was catching footballs, but Jerry's wheelhouse was negotiating big contracts. Rod felt the immense need to secure his last contract to establish financial security for himself and for his family. Nobody was listening to Rod. In a place of vulnerability, Rod turns to Jerry and says, "If you tell me to eat lima beans, I'll eat lima beans."

What Rod was saying to Jerry is, I will do whatever you tell me to do.

In life, sometimes the solution is that we get out of our own way. We need to take somebody else's hand and take our directives from someone who has trudged the path before us. I got that message from Steve and he took my hand, and with God's help and the help of our interdisciplinary program, he ended up losing 130 pounds of body fat. For Steve, it was an experience that bordered on the miraculous. ▶▶▶

You can hear Steve share his story by scanning the QR code:

198 Solving the Weight Loss Puzzle

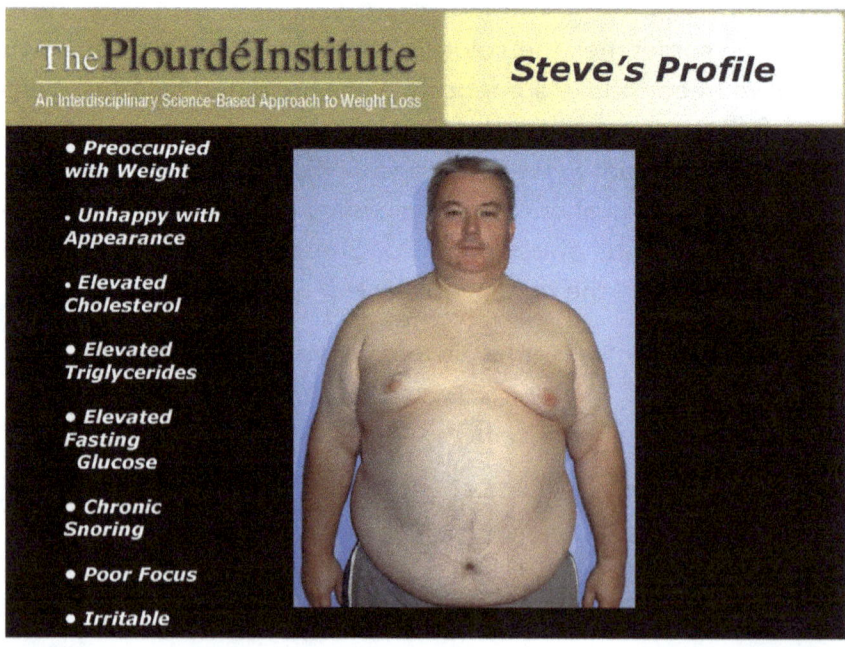

When Food is Your Drug   199

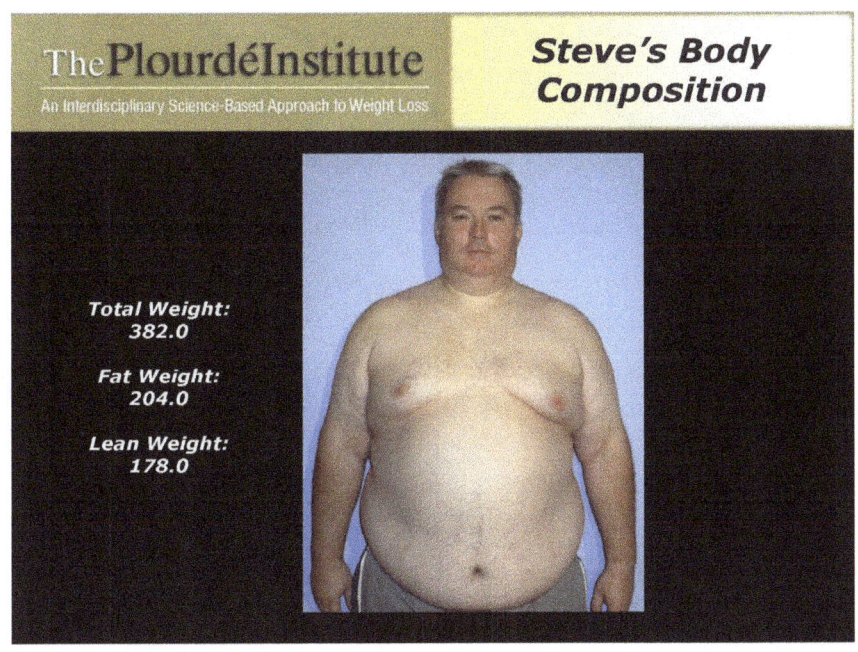

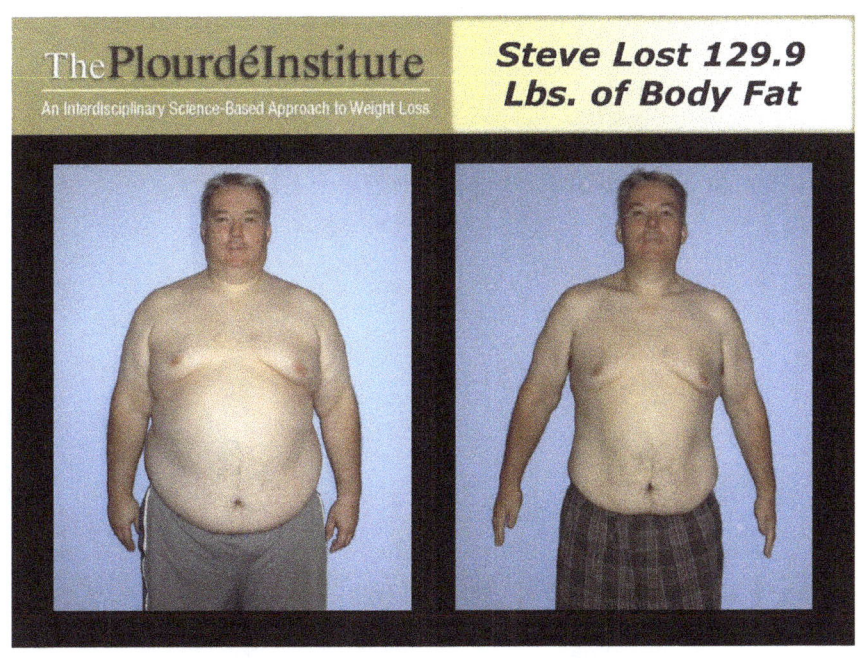

The Plourdé Institute
An Interdisciplinary Science-Based Approach to Weight Loss

Historical Evaluation of Adiposity

Name _____ Steve _____   Date _____ 10/22/2022 _____

Condition of Adiposity	Baseline	Peak	Current	Goal - 50%	Goal - 60%	Goal - 71%	Goal - 75%	Goal - 80%
Body Fat %	15.0	53.4	52.3	36.1	30.8	24.1	21.5	18.0
Fat Weight	33.0	204.0	195.0	102.0	81.6	59.2	51.0	40.8
Lean Weight	187.0	178.0	178.0	180.7	183.4	186.1	186.1	186.1
Total Weight	220.0	382.0	373.0	282.7	265.0	245.3	237.1	226.9
Age	21	44	46	46	46	46	46	46
# of Adipocytes	24.9	77.1	77.1	77.1	77.1	77.1	77.1	77.1

Fat Weight Increase of ___171.0___ lbs. = ___518.2___ %

Type of Lipogenesis =

(Type 1) Adipocyte Hypertrophy ☐

(Type 2) Adipocyte Hyperplastic Hypertrophy (Both Types) ☐

Fat Weight Reduction Goal: 93.0 lbs   =   47.7 %
                             113.4 lbs   =   58.2 %
                             135.8 lbs   =   69.7 %
                             144.0 lbs   =   73.8 %
                             154.2 lbs   =   79.1 %

Estimated Range of Reduction Phase = ___8-10___ months

Copyright © 2023 David Plourdé, Ph.D.

www.theplourdeinstitute.com
901 Warrenville Road, Suite 110, Lisle, Illinois, 60532   630.769.0776

The Plourdé Institute
An Interdisciplinary Science-Based Approach to Weight Loss

BODY COMPOSITION PROGRESS CHART

CLIENT NAME: STEVE **GOAL FAT WEIGHT: 59.2**

DATE	TOTAL WEIGHT	FAT WEIGHT	LEAN WEIGHT	FAT LOSS	% FAT LOSS	TOTAL FAT LOSS
10/22/2020	382.0	204.0	178.0			
10/22/2022	373.0	195.0	178.0	9.00	-4.4%	9.00
11/26/2022	345.5	166.2	179.3	28.77	-14.8%	37.77
1/6/2023	325.7	142.1	183.6	24.17	-14.5%	61.95
2/3/2023	314.9	130.0	184.9	12.03	-8.5%	73.98
3/3/2023	305.7	118.9	186.7	11.10	-8.5%	85.07
4/7/2023	294.8	106.9	187.9	12.00	-10.1%	97.07
6/2/2023	282.7	94.5	188.2	12.47	-11.7%	109.54
7/14/2023	278.5	89.5	189.0	5.00	-5.3%	114.54
8/25/2023	270.6	80.5	190.1	8.99	-10.0%	123.53
10/27/2023	264.7	74.1	190.6	6.41	-8.0%	129.94

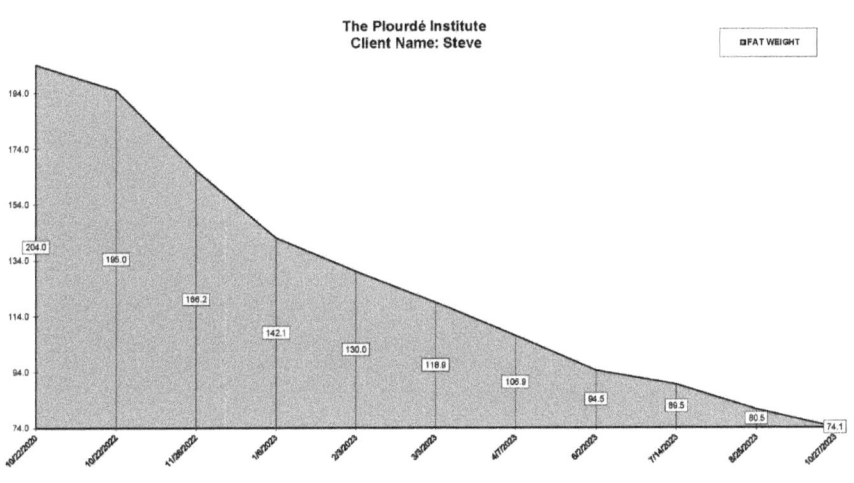

Do you see yourself in Steve's story? Can you relate with his pain? If the answer is "yes," you're not alone. Embracing the truths of the "Twelve Steps" may be the path to freedom that you've been searching for all along.

CHAPTER 14

Confessions of a Weight Loss Counselor

Confession #1: I was naïve.
I have had a front-row seat in the theater of destructive base human emotions and the self-sabotaging patterns or "games" that people engage in that torpedo their weight loss process. For many years, I was unaware of these games. Perhaps I was naïve. In my search for greater understanding, I came across a groundbreaking book by Eric Berne, M.D. entitled, *Games People Play: The Psychology of Human Relationships* (Eric Berne, 1964).

As a trained psychiatrist, he developed a theory of psychoanalysis called Transactional Analysis (TA). In this paradigm, Dr. Berne explains that there are primarily three ego states within a human being: parent, adult, and child.

In the parental ego state, we embody certain values, beliefs, and communication approaches that our parents (or parental figures) demonstrated. Sometimes, this can manifest as a "critical parent" or conversely as a "nurturing parent" in how we interact with others.

In the adult ego state, we see things objectively and analyze things rationally. We see ourselves, others, and our circumstances as they actually are.

It's been said many times that we all have a little boy or little girl inside of us. This is the child ego state. In this system of thoughts, beliefs, and emotions, we see things and operate in the mind of our inner child. Unfortunately, some of our childhood experiences may have been hurtful, abusive, or toxic because our parents or our parental figures may have been wounded themselves and unknowingly perpetuated some unhealthy patterns.

Most of us bounce from parent, adult, and child ego states unknowingly. One of the goals of Berne's system of psychoanalysis was to help people grow in their awareness of what ego state they're operating in. Subsequently, empowering the individual to choose a different ego state that enables them to live their most productive life without games or unproductive schemes, ultimately fostering an environment psychologically, emotionally, and socially where healthy relationships thrive and grow.

Berne explains in his book that the most optimum engagement between two people is from adult ego state to adult ego state because both individuals see themselves, others, and their surroundings objectively. However, sometimes our social interactions or (transactions as Berne describes them) are counterproductive because they are crossed transactions: perhaps a critical parent ego state delivers a stimulus to a child ego state causing a defensive, argumentative, or rebellious response. (Or vice versa).

Let me communicate that I am not a psychologist or a psychiatrist. I'm including this chapter because, if you're like most people, failure in weight loss has caused a lot of deep psychological and emotional pains. Sometimes, in our effort to avoid facing our failures and facing these deep pains, we engage unknowingly in unproductive and perhaps even manipulative games so as to avoid being uncomfortable.

To clarify, this is one theory of psychoanalysis and therapeutic intervention. It is one explanation of the unproductive schemes that people engage in. There are many other approaches that one can consider. To further your understanding of Dr. Berne's therapeutic model, I highly recommend that you read his book, *Games People Play*.

Confession #2: I felt ill-equipped to deal with these unhealthy tendencies and, in truth, I hated this part of my job.

That's because I didn't understand what I was observing. This was a blind spot for me. You can't solve a problem that you can't see. Therefore, for many years, I was ill-equipped to help clients effectively navigate some of their unhealthy tendencies. It took a major toll on me and in full transparency, it led to professional burnout.

One of the defining moments that helped me get a better handle on these unpleasant interactions was when I learned about the psychological paradigm of TA and, subsequently, the drama triangle. First of all, what is the drama triangle and who developed it?

The drama triangle is a model of three psychological pathologies people commonly fall into: *the victim, the rescuer, and the persecutor*. It was first coined in the 1960s by Stephen Karpman, M.D. and is explained in his book, *A Game Free Life* (Karpman, 2014).

You might be wondering why I'm including this? It's because I have observed patterns in people over the years that have confounded me. Honestly, they frustrated me, annoyed me, and drained me of my energy. More specifically, I noticed tendencies in people to sabotage themselves in their weight loss journey, not to mention creating unhealthy dynamics in the therapeutic relationship. In some cases, it derailed the efficacy of their whole process.

Let's take a closer look. The first pathology in the trifecta is called *the victim*. In this element of the paradigm, one feels powerless and unable to evoke effective change to produce a better quality of life.

They inherently feel dependent upon outward entities for their circumstances to improve. In this area of the paradigm, a person falls prey to a propensity for failing to take responsibility to make better decisions and to take the necessary actions to improve their circumstances. Fundamentally, they feel that life is happening to them, not for them. As a result, they live life in a continual state of crisis.

In psychology, there's a term called "Locus of Control Theory," which was developed in 1954 by Julian B. Rotter. The locus of control is the idea that a person either sees that they are empowered internally and able to evoke proper change and influence over the direction of their life, or instead they have an *external* locus of control where everything outwardly *is controlling them*. As you can see, the victim has a default for an external locus of control, and they are in constant stress, fear, and live in a state of perpetual powerlessness. It's an all-consuming state that precludes a person from effective weight loss and robs them of potential joy. Not good!

The second component in the trifecta of the drama triangle is *the rescuer*. This is a uniquely toxic and unhealthy pattern where a person sees themselves as a savior in somebody else's life. They have a preference for people to remain weak and dependent upon them. They can feel threatened, hurt, sad, and angry when people no longer need them. I know what you're thinking: this is really sick—and yes, it is.

Another way of looking at *the rescuer* is that they are codependent. Somehow, they thrive on or need the chaos coming from the addict and in a strange way, they are a slave to accommodating the addicted. The codependent person finds themselves walking on eggshells throughout life because they never know for sure who's showing up: is it Dr. Jekyll or Mr. Hyde? In their weakness, they seek to appease the addict by giving them the very thing that destroys them. As you can see, it's a twisted cycle.

Let me provide an example. A husband and wife embark on a weight loss journey and the husband has a profound addiction to chocolate, sugar, or some other food. After periods of abstinence, the addict finds himself irritable and unable to soothe himself. In this instance, the wife goes to the grocery store and buys him the ice cream, candy, or other food he's addicted to in order to "keep the peace." So, in her own strange way, she enables the addict and feeds the addiction, while fully aware of the complete and utter incongruency. In this case, *she* is *the rescuer.*

Thirdly, *the persecutor* is equally pathological, but in a different way. *The persecutor* is an individual who is angry, blaming outward circumstances and, commonly, their therapist, physician, weight loss counselor, personal trainer, or coach for their personal failures. I think it's appropriate, at this point, for me to mention an important observation that I have made in my career related to food addiction. There is a term in AA called the "dry drunk." It means that a person is abstaining from using, but they are not working on their interior life. They are refusing to address the psychological, emotional, and spiritual issues that are the underlying triggers to their self-medicating patterns. They are merely "white knuckling" it. They are one crisis away from sliding right back into the abyss of their addiction. You can identify these people from a mile away because they are miserable and angry because they are not using. In this context, in their frustration, they will blame their sponsor, their weight loss coach, their physician, or their spouse. This is the definition of *the persecutor.*

Regardless of which corner of the triangle a person is sitting in, here is short list of the unproductive and perhaps subconscious "games" that I have observed that are unique to the weight loss realm:

1. **This diet is too strict for me.** Instead of taking responsibility for one's addictive behaviors, the client seeks to blame the program for being too strict, and therefore sabotages the process.

2. **This meal plan is boring.** This person fails to take responsibility to expand their culinary skills. The individual seeks the same old textures and flavors instead of branching out. They don't try new recipes or seek new ways of food prep to create healthy alternatives. In passivity, they sabotage their weight loss journey.

3. **Everybody else gets to eat sugar except me.** This person plays the victim role. They fail to identify their addictive relationship with sugar and come up with reasons as to why they should use again. Inevitably, they torpedo their weight loss success.

4. **I don't have time for exercise.** Rather than acknowledge that we all have 168 hours per week and have the power to choose how we manage our time, this person plays the victim role and claims they're too busy to prioritize their health. This is an excuse.

5. **The jealousy game.** The client may harbor feelings of jealousy towards the coach. You look better than I do. I want what you have, but I can't have it, so I'm going to sabotage this process by rebelling against you.

6. **I'm too important to be accountable.** This individual hides insecurities behind a puffed-up ego. Rather than vulnerably submit to the accountability structure, they puff up their chest and act as though the program is beneath them. This is an attempt to cover up their painful insecurities and deep feelings of self-loathing.

7. **I'm going to distract you with humor or try to be your buddy while I'm noncompliant.** This person will use their pleasing personality to build rapport in an effort to distract the clinician from doing his or her job. The main goal here is to get the clinician to like them so that they avoid the inevitable accountability and perceived criticism of failing in their weight loss process.

8. **I'm too busy and important to come in for my session.** This is an avoidance behavior.

9. **It's my wife's fault.** This person seeks to blame their spouse or partner for eating in a manner that is overly tempting. Rather than take full responsibility for one's choices, they blame the other for their weight loss failure.

10. **I can't afford the program anymore.** This is a person who is not following their weight loss program and manufactures an excuse, in this case financial hardship, to escape facing their personal failure.

11. **Let me manufacture a crisis so I don't have to do this.** This is a person who is failing in their weight loss program, but rather than face the reality of their self-sabotaging behaviors, they manufacture a crisis in order to get out of their obligation and commitment.

12. **Let's talk about something else other than my weight loss program.** Distractions may include: politics, the economy, their job, their marriage, something other than the task at hand because they don't want to face the fact that they are failing to follow through.

How to Avoid the Drama Triangle

How does one avoid the triangle? I think the key element is to become psychologically, emotionally, and spiritually mature: in practical terms, it means that you *must take full responsibility for your life and your circumstances.*

If you want things to get better, and you've been living in *the victim* portion, make a real commitment to take responsibility. Take a bold step to make the decisions and to take the decisive actions needed to improve your life. You don't have to live a life shackled by feelings of powerlessness. Rather, you can move into a new realm of empowerment and personal freedom.

If your default in the trifecta is *the rescuer*, stop rescuing others when they self-sabotage. Allow people to feel and experience the consequences of their addiction, even if it means the end of a toxic relationship. Always remember people have the right to choose. Always look to empower people. If your self-worth is dependent on others, openly admit it. Are you feeling annoyed, bitter, sad, or angry when people no longer need you? Recognize it for the toxic pattern that it is and let people go. Be mindful of these tendencies and change them. If you're willing to make these changes, be prepared for deep feelings of self-respect coming your way.

If you've been defaulting to *the persecutor* role, don't blame others for your personal failures, instead, in humility, own them. Rather than be defensive about these failures and deflect, share openly and ask for help from your therapist, physician, or coach. In this way, you can shift into a new life free from bitterness, anger, and jealousy. This may be hard to imagine for the person whose tendency is to vilify others, but I've personally witnessed people pivot into a life free of these dark feelings and experience profound joy.

Confession #3: I can fall into any of the three categories of the drama triangle on any given day.

As a clinician, I can see myself as *the rescuer* looking for ways to soften the blow of consequences for non-compliant individuals. As *the persecutor*, feeling anger, frustration, or annoyance, I can look for ways to blame others for my lack of boundaries with clients. As *the victim*, I can be overwhelmed by a sense of powerlessness when I don't understand how to solve a problem in my business or my personal life. An interesting point I want to make is that now, after having learned about the drama triangle, when I see these tendencies in myself, I can quickly course correct. This has been an invaluable insight and has improved the quality of my mental and emotional health, and I believe it can for you, too.

Now, here are some lessons that I share with my clients and now have the privilege of sharing with you. If you're feeling powerless and weak, you need to work for solutions and commit to make the bold moves to course correct your life psychologically, emotionally, physically, relationally, financially, and professionally. Are you blaming others? Are you annoyed, frustrated, or bitter? You need to set better boundaries in your life. In these instances, you need to learn how to say "no," as Stephen Covey wrote in his book *The Seven Habits of Highly Effective People* (Covey, 2004). As he explains in his "Time Management Matrix," you need to say no to the proximate, the pressing, and the popular and say yes to life-building disciplines. He taught that it is much easier to say no to the unimportant and urgent interruptions of life when you have a big enough and bright enough burning "yes." In this case, your "yes" is related to the prioritization of your own self-care. You are fully responsible for your circumstances. What changes can you make right now to make things better for yourself?

Let me say it again, these psychological patterns are a problem for many people. Unaware of these pathologies, people will limp along, coping in an unhealthy manner with the conflicts that emerge in their own minds and in the relationships they have with those around them. Don't you think it's time for us to turn the lights on and avoid these common pitfalls?

The three big ideas in this chapter are to be aware of your ego states, the unconscious games that you may have played or are playing in your weight loss journey, and the potential pitfalls of the drama triangle.

Originally, I wasn't sure if I would include this chapter in the book, but I'm glad that I did. My own lack of awareness of these ideas resulted in a lot of pain in my life, both professionally and personally. With greater awareness of these principles, not only will you have more success in your weight loss effort, but you'll also maintain much better mental and emotional health.

CHAPTER 15

The Power of Faith

Could it be that the freedom, better health, joy, and self-respect that you are so diligently seeking will come not by working harder but, rather, through faith? Strangely, you may find that the answer to this question is yes!

What is Faith?
Faith is defined in the book of Hebrews in the Bible. "Now faith is the substance of things hoped for, the evidence of things not seen. (Hebrews 11:1 NKJV)

Faith is practically a palpable property. When you have it you know it, and you can just about reach out and touch it.

▶▶▶ One of my first experiences with faith occurred, surprisingly, after suffering a catastrophic elbow injury. When I was a freshman in high school, I was recruited to the wrestling team. I had really good upper body strength and the coaches recognized it, so they persuaded me to join the team. It wasn't my forte, and I had not trained in wrestling prior to this. I was a starter on the freshman wrestling team in the 145-pound weight class, but I had difficulty making weight, so I would wear a sauna suit to sweat excessively and do strenuous exercise to lose weight.

One evening, in an effort to cut weight for my quad meet the next day, I was playing one-on-one basketball in my sauna suit with my friend Kraig. While we were playing, he accidentally tripped me as I was going for a layup. Falling from close to the rim level, I landed on the concrete driveway squarely on my left elbow. It swelled immediately to two to three times its normal size and I was in a lot of pain. When I showed up at Mr. Carey's training room the next day prior to the quad meet, he taped my elbow extensively and gave me the okay to wrestle.

Well, things didn't go very well. In my match with a very competitive wrestler from Main West High School, we were in a stalemate and went to the ground. That's when the trouble hit. My elbow snapped off backward. It was a grotesque sight. My brother, Bill, came quickly to the high school gym as the ambulance was taking me to the ER. The growth plate was broken off and the ulnar nerve had been crushed. Within a couple of days, I had reconstructive surgery that required the insertion of pins to reattach the growth plate to my elbow. This is the "funny bone" that tingles when you hit it. Despite the successful surgery, I had no feeling from my elbow all the way to the tips of my fingers for a few months.

Dr. O'Neill was a very skilled orthopedic surgeon, but unfortunately, he gave me no input for my prognosis. I was completely in the dark as to the nature of how my elbow would recover. As an insecure freshman in high school, I was devastated.

My unspoken dream was to become the strongest kid in the state of Illinois. I could not exercise for months, and I lay awake sleepless

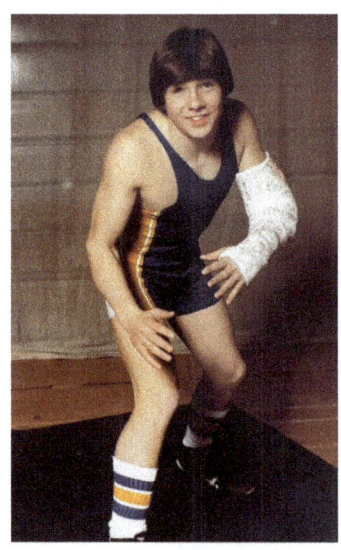

Credit: Personal Photo

every night because I was so distraught that my dream of becoming a state champion competitive powerlifter had died.

The day finally came when my dad picked me up from Lyons Township High School in Western Springs, Illinois, to take me to Dr. O'Neil's office. This was the moment I had been anxiously awaiting for months: he would take out the pins from my elbow and I would learn what my fate was.

Something that's true is that my dad, William M. Plourdé ("Big Bill" as my family called him), knew me better than I knew myself. He knew how much I had been struggling. As I sat anxiously waiting to hear from the physician about what was up ahead, my dad spoke up and said, "Go ahead and ask the doctor your question."

I choked up as I asked, "Will I ever be able to lift weights again?" I was dreading his answer.

Dr. O'Neill smirked and said, "You could lift weights today if you wanted to. I don't know why you would want to do that, though."

My dad quietly smiled at me and winked. I knew what that meant: we weren't going back to the high school; we were going straight home.

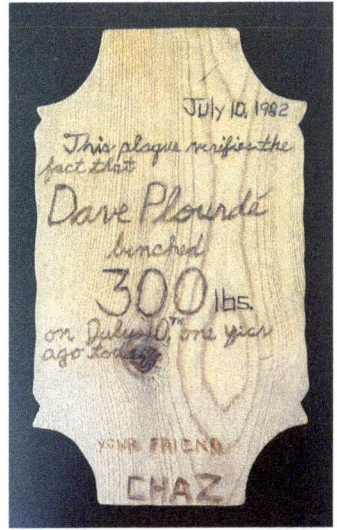

With my dad's help, I did my first bench press that day, lifting the bar off the rack with two hands on the left and then my right hand on the right. Let me just add that I had about a one-inch range of motion with my left elbow at this point. It wasn't pretty and I had a very long way to go.

This is where faith came in for me in such a real way. Once the physician told me I could lift weights, I feverishly

Credit: Personal Photo

and carefully plotted my training. Within less than six months, I went on to bench press 300 pounds. It was really a miracle. One of my dear friends, Charlie Galanti (a.k.a. Chaz) made a plaque for me, signifying this momentous outcome. I was so touched by Charlie's compassion for me and his thoughtfulness.

As a young person, I realized I had a knack for training. I had essentially a photographic memory for everything I ever did with my weight training and what the outcomes were. By the time I was a senior in high school, without using anabolic steroids, I bench-pressed nearly 500 pounds and went on to become a Chicagoland High School Champion and Best Lifter. I later became Teenage State Champion and Best Lifter, as well as Junior State Champion, setting numerous state records. All of this occurred while I was under the tutelage of former World Champion and author Mr. Bill Seno. I can never thank him enough for all of his sacrifices. I'll explain later in this chapter how faith played a significant role in my recovery. ▶▶▶

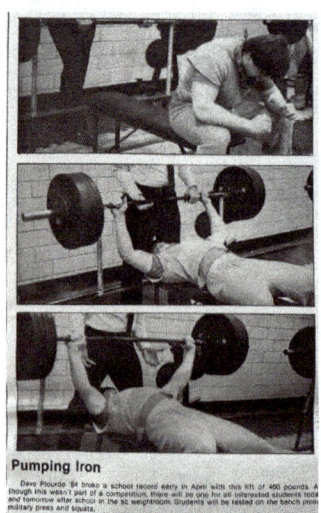

Credit: Lyons Township High School Newspaper "The Lion"

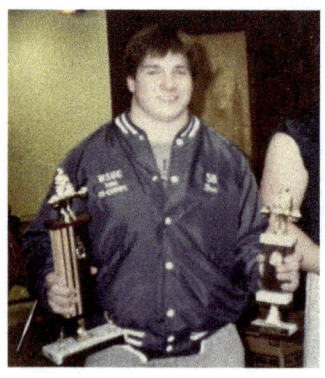

Credit: Family photo

Now, let's look further into faith. Paul wrote in the New Testament, "Consequently, faith comes from hearing the message, and the message is heard through the word about Christ." (Romans 10:17 NIV)

In other words, faith comes through your ears. The book of Genesis says that

God spoke creation into existence. Back in Romans it says, "If you declare with your mouth, 'Jesus is Lord,' and believe in your heart that God raised him from the dead, you will be saved. For it is with your heart that you believe and are justified, and it is with your mouth that you profess your faith and are saved." (Romans 10:9-10 NIV)

The book of Proverbs says the tongue has the power of both life and death. Here we see very clearly that spoken words are heard and have great power; perhaps a level of power you can't even imagine.

▶▶▶ This is where it gets personal for me: after recovering from my catastrophic elbow injury, I became a disciplined goal-setter. I learned this discipline from my big brother Bill (who my family called "Little Bill"), who was a mentor and a source of continual encouragement for me.

I grew up in a middle-class family in Hinsdale, Illinois. Our family didn't have a lot of money, but we had a nice house with an unfinished basement. We had a shower in the basement and that was where the laundry room was. This was my preferred place to get ready for school.

In the basement, my dad had placed an enormous chalkboard on the concrete wall. I developed a habit of writing down my bench press goals on this chalkboard in extraordinarily large numerals. Every week I would write down my bench press goal. As I mentioned earlier, at the end of my freshman year of high school after the elbow injury, I bench pressed 300 pounds. By the end of my senior year, I was able to bench press 460 pounds. After I had believed in the depth of my being that my dream of being a state champion was dead, my dream was resurrected *by faith.*

During my senior year, I would write down my goal every week. The first week it was 410. The second week it was 415, and all the way up to 460. You get the picture.

This is where I accidentally tripped over a principle of faith: I would fix my eyes on that number on the chalkboard and with complete psychological, emotional, and verbal intensity, I would say, "YES!!!!" I accompanied this with a power move, such as a karate chop. I know this sounds silly, but it actually worked. The idea that I could accomplish something that was seemingly impossible after having such a serious injury truly was a miracle for me. I BELIEVED. ▶▶▶

I know I said it at the outset of the chapter, but I'm going to say it again: faith is the substance (it's practically palpable, and you know it when you have it) of things hoped for; it is the evidence of things we can't see. So, my hope is that you don't have to suffer a catastrophic injury to find your own faith. If I can learn how to harness the power of faith, so can you!

How Does Faith Apply to Your Weight Loss Journey?

Well, in the words of Henry Ford, "Whether you think you can, or you think you can't—you're right." You *must* believe. A strange fact here is that you can activate your faith with your mouth just as I stumbled across this principle as a freshman in high school. You can apply this principle in your own life here and now, and with advanced physical science, an understanding of psychology, and the power of faith, you can overcome your lifelong struggle, just as the thousands of men and women I have coached have done before you. If they can succeed, why not you? Why not now?

CHAPTER 16

The Keys to Long Term Weight Loss Success

You may have heard, or even personally experienced, just how pitiful long-term weight loss statistics really are. Sadly, this is true, but it doesn't have to be this way. This chapter is designed to help you identify and avoid common stumbling blocks to long-term success.

As we begin this chapter, I'd like to discuss a scientific journal article that sheds light on the different types of weight loss follow up. The landmark study by Ayyad and Anderson published in 2000, entitled "Long-term efficacy of dietary treatment of obesity: A systematic review of studies published between 1931 and 1999" (Ayyad, 2000), may be the most comprehensive analysis of long-term weight loss ever conducted.

Let's take a look at that study: The authors identified 898 papers published on the subject of weight loss between 1931 and 1999. Of the 898 papers, only seventeen papers met their inclusion criteria, which was the following:

> **First**: They selected papers that dealt exclusively with adults.
>
> **Second**: The follow up period for weight loss maintenance was for at least three years or more.
>
> **Third**: Because all of the papers had different definitions of weight loss success, the authors of this study created a standard definition which was the following:

Participants that maintained their weight loss or had additional weight loss at the three year mark were considered successful.

Fourth: The total number of subjects that met this inclusion criteria among the seventeen papers was 2,131. This was the study group.

Among the seventeen papers, there were three types of weight loss follow-up:

- Passive
- Active
- Active and Therapeutic

The passive follow-up was really no follow up at all. This approach lacked structure, accountability, and was disorganized. Only 10 percent of the participants in this group maintained their weight loss within the three-year period. In other words, 90 percent of the passive follow up group regained their weight.

The second type of follow-up was active. This group was subjected to a consistent follow-up that was organized and provided accountability with weight loss maintenance. Nineteen percent of the participants in the Active group maintained their weight loss at the three year mark, but 81 percent of the subjects regained their weight within the three year period.

The third type of follow-up was active *and* therapeutic. This type of follow-up included all of the accountability, organization, and structure as the active follow-up, but also included group therapy. Groups such as these address the psychological and emotional aspects of eating behavior. As you might have expected, the results were better for this group. Twenty-seven percent of the active and therapeutic group maintained their weight loss at the three year period.

So, we can conclude that the active and therapeutic follow up group was nearly three times more likely to maintain their weight loss at the three year mark than the passive group. However, when you look at the data in its entirety, the overall rate of success is certainly less than inspiring.

As a scientist, from the very outset, it has been my goal to develop a highly effective, science-based approach to weight loss with the ultimate purpose of liberating people from this lifelong, preoccupying problem.

A number of years ago, I began to include the presentation of the Ayyad and Anderson study on long-term weight loss. I thought to myself, "Surely if I present this information, people will choose to remain in an active and therapeutic follow up." I was sorely disappointed. So, I went back through all the data I had accumulated and the observations of the stages of thousands of subjects that had gone through the weight loss process. I wanted to see if there were specific patterns to shed light on why people relapsed.

The following is the essence of that work:

Somehow, a person who has been struggling with the pain of unsuccessful weight loss finds THE PLOURDE METHOD℠. At the outset of their journey, our interdisciplinary science-based METHOD is carefully explained. The person understands the METHOD and feels very hopeful. This hopefulness translates to motivation and the motivation manifests in a very high rate of compliance.

An important detail to know about the inclusion criteria of my original research was that subjects were clinically overweight and had to be at or near their highest body fat weight in their lifetime and had relatively normal body fat levels at the baseline of physical maturity.

When our private clients meet our compliance criteria, body fat weight loss occurs at a mathematically linear rate, within the range of 10 to 20 percent per month, every month. This unusual rate of progress results in greater hopefulness, motivation, and continued compliance. Eventually, the person approaches a natural biological plateau in body fat weight loss:

- For women, the plateau occurs somewhere between 61 and 73 percent from peak body fat weight.
- For men, the plateau occurs somewhere between 71 and 80 percent from peak body fat weight.

(As a reminder, these statistics displayed above reflect the implementation of the full breadth of intellectual property and trade secrets of my METHOD reserved for private clients. The content that I am sharing in this book may result in greater than 50 percent body fat weight loss from your peak body fat weight.)

It has been my observation that as a person approaches this natural biological plateau, their prior confusion is replaced with clarity. Their anger is replaced with self-respect. Instead of feeling shame and self-loathing, one feels accomplished. Joyfulness in one's masculinity or femininity may be re-established. The over-all state could be described as euphoric.

But it's in this state of euphoria that people are often deceived. They often feel and perceive as though they've been cured. But unfortunately, this is not the case. As we spoke about in the addiction chapter, the process of weight loss can be likened to a sobriety journey, such as recovery from alcoholism. When a person hits "bottom" and decides to change their life, they may find themselves going to AA, getting a sponsor, and working the "Twelve Steps." Through a process of personal accountability, personal growth, and major behavioral change, a person gets sober. Once sober, participants often feel free of the pain of their addictive behavior and find themselves feeling euphoric.

It's my opinion that the key to long-term sobriety and *long-term weight loss success is found in how a person responds to their absence of pain. If a person remains humble and teachable in their newly-found freedom, remains accountable, and does not relent in their quest for continual personal growth, then they will have the best chance of remaining successful.*

Disciplines of personal growth might include solitude, meditation, journaling, and prayer. Other disciplines such as eating healthy, exercise, expanding one's emotional intelligence, growing in spirituality, and mindfulness of one's psychology of behavior are also very helpful. Frequent accountability and deep personal growth are fixtures in this person's life.

Now, the *alternative response* to the absence of pain in this newly-found freedom is to become *overconfident, perhaps even cocky*, in one's sobriety or weight loss success. A person might say to themselves, "I'm cured. I no longer need to be accountable because I've got this figured out. This accountability stuff is overrated. I've got it from here on out."

Well, eventually, a crisis comes along: a job change, a problem with a child, a divorce, or the death of a loved one. Because this person is not involved in deep personal growth and in regular accountability, they default back to unhealthy coping patterns and fall headlong into addictive behavior. This is because *they failed to internalize the importance of remaining humble and teachable.* They were unable, or perhaps unwilling, to recognize the importance of accountability and deep personal growth as prerequisites of long-term sobriety or weight loss success.

As the study showed, the three year period is a significant demarcation, and unfortunately, most people fail to internalize these realities and gain their weight back. Let me confess that this has always been a sad and difficult pill for me to swallow as a clinician. It is always my hope for people to see the light of these truths. The fullness of time always reveals who was truly receptive and who wasn't.

As I have mentioned many times, pain is strangely a very important piece in the weight loss puzzle: the higher the pain level—the more receptive the person is to change.

Over the years, as I've documented human behavior, I have also studied the Bible. A passage that may offer insight on the idea of a person's receptivity is found in the Gospel of Mark chapter 4. It is also known as the "Parable of the Soil." Jesus describes four soil types:

> The Path—hard and impenetrable
>
> The Rocky Soil—shallow
>
> The Weedy Soil—chock filled with weeds
>
> The Good Soil—watered, weeded, receptive, and ultimately fruitful

We will discuss this further after you have had the chance to read the Parable for yourself:

> *Again Jesus began to teach by the lake. The crowd that gathered around him was so large that he got into a boat and sat in it out on the lake, while all the people were along the shore at the water's edge. He taught them many things by parables, and in his teaching said: "Listen! A farmer went out to sow his seed. As he was scattering the seed, some fell along the path, and*

the birds came and ate it up. Some fell on rocky places, where it did not have much soil. It sprang up quickly, because the soil was shallow. But when the sun came up, the plants were scorched, and they withered because they had no root. Other seed fell among thorns, which grew up and choked the plants, so that they did not bear grain. Still other seed fell on good soil. It came up, grew and produced a crop, some multiplying thirty, sixty, or even a hundred times.

Then Jesus said, 'He who has ears to hear, let him hear."

When he was alone, the Twelve and the others around him asked him about the parables. He told them, "The secret of the kingdom of God has been given to you. But to those on the outside everything is said in parables so that, 'they may be ever seeing but never perceiving, and ever hearing but never understanding;otherwise they might turn and be forgiven!'

Then Jesus said to them, "Don't you understand this parable? How then will you understand any parable? The farmer sows the word. Some people are like seed along the path, where the word is sown. As soon as they hear it, Satan comes and takes away the word that was sown in them. Others, like seed sown on rocky places, hear the word and at once receive it with joy. But since they have no root, they last only a short time. When trouble or persecution comes because of the word, they quickly fall away. Still others, like seed sown among thorns, hear the word; but the worries of this life, the deceitfulness of wealth and the desires for other things come in and choke the word, making it unfruitful. Others, like seed sown on good soil, hear the word, accept it, and produce a crop—thirty, sixty or even a hundred times what was sown. (Mark 4:1-20 NIV)

In the first soil type, a person hears the secret of the Kingdom of Heaven but they don't understand it and Satan steals the Word from the person's mind, rendering it unfruitful. In the second soil type, the Rocky Soil, this represents a person who has a shallow commitment to the idea, ultimately rendering the idea unproductive. The third soil type, the Weedy Soil, represents a person who is stressed out, worried about money, or preoccupied by competing desires. As a result, they lack bandwidth and the idea is powerless. The fourth soil is called the Good Soil. This represents a scenario where the person **hears** the idea, **understands** it, and **applies** it, thus experiencing the full power of the idea.

I am in no way suggesting that THE PLOURDE METHOD℠ in any way should be compared to the importance of the salvation message of the Bible. I'm simply sharing the parallel that I have seen in my career demonstrating differences in how people respond to new learning and how that translates to the impact the idea has on a person's life. I have seen that when I present our scientific METHOD to a prospective new client, there are really only four possible responses:

1. They don't understand it.
2. They have a shallow commitment to the idea.
3. They're stressed out or preoccupied with competing desires and lack bandwidth.
4. They hear it, accept it, and apply it, resulting in significant body fat weight loss.

So, let me circle the wagons. As I've mentioned, when people have major weight loss success, they often feel euphoric and fall prey to the deception that they're cured and don't need further accountability.

This response may be a reflection of the Rocky Soil, showing that in the fullness of time their commitment may have been shallow. Perhaps they were over confident in their absence of pain, eventually regaining all of their weight. Regardless of whether a person is lacking aptitude, shallow in their commitment, or stressed out and overwhelmed, the idea doesn't take. Only the person who hears, accepts, and applies the given idea will enjoy long-term benefits and the full power of that idea.

Sadly, few people actually do this.

I've found it difficult to wrap my mind around the fact that most people will probably not "get it." I have had the privilege of serving many people who were members of AA and have remained sober for more than twenty-plus years. When I ask them what percentage of people who get sober remain sober, their answer is: about 5 percent. So, whether the object of dependency is food, alcohol, or something else, only in the fullness of time will we know who internalized the key principles and who didn't.

> **The keys to long-term weight loss success are:**
> **Remain humble—don't get cocky.**
> **Remain accountable.**

In conclusion, don't be fooled by the euphoria that comes with major weight loss success and sobriety. As the statistics indicate, sadly, most people bow out after their initial weight loss experience. At Plourdé, for those who do remain in an active and therapeutic follow-up, the vast majority of them maintain their weight loss. I hope you, too, recognize the importance of these principles in your weight loss journey and enjoy long-lasting success.

CHAPTER 17

A Personal Invitation from Dr. Plourdé

I want to personally commend you for making the sacrifice to set aside your valuable time to read this book. If you're reading this, I can tell you with certainty that throughout this journey so far, you have demonstrated faith, humility, and courage. These are fundamental keys to solving your weight loss puzzle.

Furthermore, I don't take your sacrifices lightly, and I thoroughly appreciate your openness to the messages that I have written in this book.

Where do we go from here?

If you apply the principles that I have laid out for you, you may accomplish a 50 percent reduction from your peak body fat weight. From the very beginning, I made it clear that the contents of this book could help you to replace your pain and help you come into a new life of freedom, better health, joy, and self-respect. This is my hope and prayer for you.

Additional Resources/ Next Steps

To further assist you, I have made even more content available to you:

- **Our website—ThePlourdeMethod.com**

    Find additional complimentary resources regarding meal plans, science-based exercise tips, as well as other helpful tools. This will include:

- **An online food and exercise tracker along with a journal** to record your foods, fluids, and eating behaviors, as well as a section to unpackage incongruent thoughts and feelings that have been notorious in tripping you up in past weight loss efforts.

- **A body fat weight loss calculator** that can help you *have realistic expectations* for how much body fat weight loss is physiologically possible for you and how long it will take.

    Available with a subscription (Coming in 2025):

- **Video curriculum where I systematically and compassionately teach you on a deeper level** about the principles of THE PLOURDE METHOD℠ .

- Proprietary Recipe Library backed by metabolic research to guarantee no suppression in the fat cell.

- Available for purchase: on-plan, Plourdé Nutrition brand supplements free of insidious sugars and starches.

- Options for one-on-one coaching packages

If you would like to become a private client of The Plourdé Institute, go to the website ThePlourdeMethod.com or call our 24/7 intake department at 844-756-8733 for more information.

From the bottom of my heart, it has been a pleasure to share these ideas with you: the hero of our story! Please keep us posted with your weight loss progress on social media (tag us on Instagram: @theplourdemethod, on Facebook: The Plourde Method, and use the hashtags #ThePlourdeMethod and #SolvingTheWeightLossPuzzle.

I wish you all the best on your journey toward better health, joy, and self-respect!

Sincerely,
David B. Plourdé, Ph.D.

Scan this QR Code to be directed to ThePlourdeMethod.com.

Acknowledgments

I first must thank my parents, Bill and Doris Plourdé. My father was a renaissance man; he was good at everything. Growing up, he was a talented baseball player and was recruited to the Chicago Cubs farm system in the 1950s. He had the privilege of playing with baseball legend Ernie Banks. After suffering a career-ending elbow injury, he had to put his dream of playing in the major leagues on the shelf. He transferred his passion for competitive sports to golf and became a very successful player, winning an amateur golf championship just before he passed away from cancer in 2001. He was a natural born salesman, a good cook, and had an amazing ability to connect with others. My father was a man's man and knew me better than I knew myself. It was through his patience, love, and wisdom that he helped me become the man that I am. I wish I were half the man that my father was.

My mom, Doris Plourdé, is a beautiful human being inside and out. After having two kids, my sister Loree and brother Bill, she had always wanted a third child. After a seven-year gap, along came me—the bonus child! She loved the name David and that was the name they agreed upon for me. As the baby of the family, I was given a lot of attention and nurturing from the family. This year she turns ninety, and she still exudes an incredible positive loving energy. She is the eternal optimist and lights up the room wherever she is. Her warmth, love, and positivity have been anchors for me throughout my life. My parents' unconditional love, support, and countless sacrifices shaped me to become the person writing this book. I am eternally grateful to them.

My sister, Loree, paved the way for my brother Bill and me. A great big sister, she's always been there for me. As you found out, a gift from her is one of the reasons this book exists. She has been a constant source of support and encouragement in my life.

Of course, none of the content of this book would have ever been created if it weren't for my team of field experts: Kathleen Rourke, Ph.D.; Glenn Town, Ph.D.; Brad Lindell, Ph.D.; Beverly Rubik, Ph.D.; and Carol Barrett, Ph.D. They thoughtfully guided me in all of the phases of my work. They encouraged me and reassured me every step of the way. Their insight and wisdom helped me to avoid many pitfalls along the journey. Thank you all!

I also want to thank my team of unbiased biomedical students and staff. They were immensely helpful in bettering our understanding of imperceptible chemical qualities in food, fluids, and products, and their implications on Hormone-Sensitive Lipase function in the human fat cell. Over the decades of our data collection and documentation, these dedicated individuals were behind the scenes and I could never have accomplished my research objectives without their faithful support. Thank you all from the bottom of my heart.

Additionally, I want to thank my publishing team members at the Steve Harrison Group and additional consultants: Lynn Tramonte, Cristina Smith, Valerie Costas, Christy Day, Michael Levin, and Allan Haggar, M.D.. Thank you for sharing your wisdom, expertise, and time to help make my manuscript the best it could possibly be.

I want to thank my daughters Sophia Mueller, Briana Plourdé, Venessa Plourdé, and Alana Plourdé. Sophia invested countless hours of administrative support in the creation of this book and stepped up to lead our clients while I was focusing on writing. Briana was particularly helpful in the creation of the technical diagrams featured throughout this book. Thank you to Venessa for her continual encouragement and prayers. Alana has supported our business with her incredible video editing skills that you have seen in some of the videos displayed throughout this book. Thank you all so much! I love you!

Last but not least, I want to thank my wife, Tiffany Plourdé. She has stood by me in the many moments when I doubted myself and wanted to quit this project. She believed in me. I also have her to thank for her countless hours of editing and her assistance in refining the manuscript. She prayed for me and lovingly supported me through much of my arduous journey. I could never have done this without you. Thank you!

Bibliography

Ayyad, C. & Andersen, T. 2000. "Long-term efficacy of dietary treatment of obesity: A systematic review of studies published between 1931 and 1999." *Obesity Reviews* 113-119.

Created in BioRender. Plourde, D., Plourde, B. (2024) BioRender.com/m65f625

Created in BioRender. Plourde, D., Plourde, B. (2024) BioRender.com/b68u802

Created in BioRender. Plourde, D., Plourde, B. (2024) BioRender.com/d16y439

Created in BioRender. Plourde, D., Plourde, B. (2024) BioRender.com/j68y821

Created in BioRender. Plourde, D., Plourde, B. (2024) BioRender.com/f35o957

Borg, Gunnar. 1998. "Borg's perceived exertion and pain scales." *Human Kinetics.*

n.d. *Cambridge Business English Dictionary website s.v. "accountability".* Accessed August 13, 2024. https://dictionary.cambridge.org/us/dictionary/english/accountability.

Chhabra, Neeta. 2020. *Slideshare.* 23 April. Accessed 02 28, 2024. www.slideshare.net/neetachhabra/development-of-foregut-232501476.

Covey, Stephen R. 2004. *The 7 Habits of Highly Effective People: Powerful Lessons in Personal Change.* 15. New York: Free Press.

1996. *Jerry Maguire.* Directed by Cameron Crowe. Produced by TriStar Pictures.

n.d. *Dictionary Merriam-Webster.com s.v. "account".* Accessed August 13, 2024. https://www.merriam-webster.com/dictionary/account.

Eric Berne, M.D. 1964. *Games People Play: The Psychology of Human Relationships.* Grove Press.

2024. "Exerise Physiology & Human Performance." *Texas A&M University —Central Texas.* Accessed 08 13, 2024. https://www.tamuct.edu/degrees/undergraduate/exercise-physiology.html.

Foster, Michelle T., and Michael J. Pagliassotti. 2012. ""Metabolic alterations following visceral fat removal and expansion: Beyond anatomic location"." *Adipocyte col. 1,4* 192-199.

Hirsch, Dr. Jules M. 1971. "Adipose Cellularity in Relation to Human Obesity."

2023. "http://fis.fda.gov." *FDA Adverse Events Reporting System (FAERS) Public Dashboard.* 31 December. Accessed 2 28, 2024. https://fis.fda.gov/sense/app/95239e26-e0be-42d9-a960-9a5f7f1c25ee/sheet/45beeb74-30ab-46be-8267-5756582633b4/state/analysis.

2023. "https://fis.fda.gov." *FDA Adverse Events Reporting System (FAERS) Public Dashboard.* 31 December. Accessed February 28, 2024. https://fis.fda.gov/sense/app/95239e26-e0be-42d9-a960-9a5f7f1c25ee/sheet/45beeb74-30ab-46be-8267-5756582633b4/state/analysis.

Jensterle M, Ferjan S, Ležaič L, Sočan A, Goričar K, Zaletel K, Janez A. 2023. ""Semaglutide delays 4-hour gastric emptying in women with polycystic ovary syndrome and obesity"." *Diabetes, obesity & metabolism.*

Kapit, Wynn and Elson, Lawrence M. 1993. *The Anatomy Coloring Book, Second Edition.* HarperCollins.

Kapit, Wynn, Robert L. Macey, and Esmail Meisami. 1987. *The Physiology Coloring Book.* New York: HarperCollins.

Karpman M.D., Stephen B. 2014. *A Game Free Life - The definitive book on the Drama Triangle and Compassion Triangle by the originator and author.* San Francisco: Drama Triangle Publications.

Livingston, E., Sebastian, J., Huerta, S., Yip, I., & Heber, D. 2001. "Bio-exponential Model for Predicting Weight-Loss after Gastric Surgery for Obesity." *Journal of Surgical Research* 216-224.

Mayo Clinic Staff. 2022. *Mayo Clinic.* 12 10. Accessed 02 24, 2024. www.mayoclinic.org/healthy-lifestyle/nutrition-and-healthy-eating/in-depth/water/art-20044256.

Roscoe, Wendi A. 2019. *Human Biology, Anatomy & Physiology for the Health Sciences, 2nd Edition.* Top Hat.

1986. *Top Gun.* Directed by Tony Scott. Performed by James Tolkan.

www.aa.org. 1952, 1953, 1981. "Alcoholics Anonymous®." *www.aa.org.* Accessed 02 28, 2024. www.aa.org/the-twelve-steps.

About The Author

Dr. David Plourdé holds a Ph.D. in sciences with concentrations in human nutrition and exercise physiology from Union Institute and University. Prior to receiving his doctoral science credentials, Plourdé was a social worker with a background in food addiction recovery, graduating with a Bachelor of Arts degree from the University of Wisconsin-Whitewater. As a follower of Jesus Christ, Dr. Plourdé's original intention was to continue his studies in seminary after completing his undergraduate degree. However, that all changed after he experienced a spiritual awakening, which led him to a new calling and direction for his life in science.

Dr. Plourdé has been studying human nutrition, chemistry, metabolic research, exercise physiology, muscle metabolism, body composition science, the psychology of eating behavior, and food addiction recovery in a laboratory setting for thirty-three years (over 85,000 clinical hours).

Thousands of overweight men and women (from California to New York, Minnesota to South Florida) have successfully lost significant and life changing body fat weight through his scientific weight loss method. With the help of a team of field experts, Dr. Plourdé relentlessly pursued three primary objectives in his research:

1. To develop a noninvasive technique to monitor the enzyme Hormone-Sensitive Lipase (HSL), an enzyme responsible for regulating the weight of each individual fat cell.
2. To pioneer an interdisciplinary scientific method (which

eventually became THE PLOURDE METHOD℠) to FULLY control the HSL enzyme, reducing fat cell weight and body fat levels in an entirely predictable and reproducible fashion.

3. To select and establish a statistical tool to predict when the brain perceives a threat from fat cells getting too small, resulting in a biological plateau in weight loss. This is similar to how a yellow light comes on in your car's dashboard indicating you are critically low on fuel.

These objectives were accomplished after implementing three human trials and answering to the Institutional Review Board of Union Institute and University. This requirement is a safeguard for the safe and ethical treatment of human subjects in research. He tracked 308 adult, overweight, human subjects, divided among three trials over many years—with seven-day-a-week doctor-patient interaction.

The result of this extensive research, trials, and refinements is called THE PLOURDE METHOD℠. It has become *the road map* to successfully navigate your weight loss journey, drawn from decades of clinical experience by the nation's leader in science-based weight loss.

www.ingramcontent.com/pod-product-compliance
Lightning Source LLC
Chambersburg PA
CBHW070617030426
42337CB00020B/3832